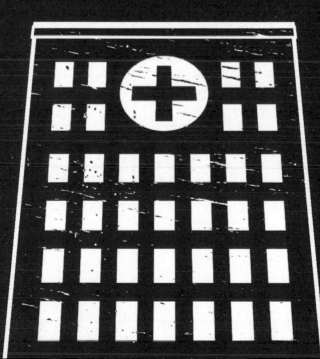

STRUCTURES OF
INDIFFERENCE

STRUCTURES OF
INDIFFERENCE

An Indigenous Life and Death in a Canadian City

MARY JANE LOGAN McCALLUM AND ADELE PERRY

UNIVERSITY OF MANITOBA PRESS

Structures of Indifference: An Indigenous Life
and Death in a Canadian City
© Mary Jane Logan McCallum and Adele Perry 2018

22   21   20   19   3   4   5   6

University of Manitoba Press
Winnipeg, Manitoba, Canada
Treaty 1 Territory
uofmpress.ca

Cataloguing data available from Library and Archives Canada
ISBN 978-0-88755-835-1 (PAPER)
ISBN 978-0-88755-573-2 (PDF)
ISBN 978-0-88755-571-8 (EPUB)

Cover design by Mike Carroll
Interior design by Jess Koroscil

Printed in Canada

All royalties from the sale of this book will be donated to support
the programs of Ka Ni Kanichihk Inc.

The University of Manitoba Press acknowledges the financial
support for its publication program provided by the Government
of Canada through the Canada Book Fund, the Canada Council
for the Arts, the Manitoba Department of Sport, Culture,
and Heritage, the Manitoba Arts Council, and
the Manitoba Book Publishing Tax Credit.

Funded by the Government of Canada   Canadä

CONTENTS

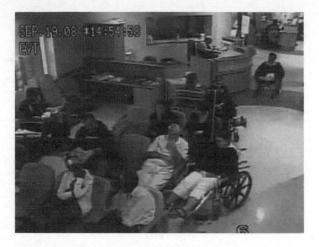

Figure 1. Still image from the HSC surveillance video camera that recorded Brian Sinclair's arrival at the Emergency Department triage desk at 2:54 p.m. on 19 September 2008. There is approximately 500 hours of security camera footage of the thirty-four hours Sinclair spent in the HSC Emergency waiting room.

INTRODUCTION
THIRTY-FOUR HOURS

THIS BOOK IS ABOUT AN Indigenous life and death in a Canadian city, and what it reveals about the ongoing history of colonialism and Indigenous people's relationship to it. At the core of this story are thirty-four hours that passed in September 2008. During that day and a half, Brian Sinclair, a middle-aged, non-status Anishinaabe resident of Winnipeg, Manitoba's capital city, wheeled himself into the emergency room of the Health Sciences Centre (HSC), the city's major downtown hospital, was left untreated and unattended to, and ultimately passed away from an easily treatable infection. This, we argue, reflects a particular structure of indifference born of and maintained by colonialism, and one that can best be understood by situating this particular Indigenous life and death within their historical context.

The book builds on Mary Jane Logan McCallum's work with the Brian Sinclair Working Group (BSWG). Led by Dr. Barry Lavallee, physician and educator; Emily Hill, lawyer with Aboriginal

Legal Services; Dr. Annette Browne, professor at the School of Nursing, University of British Columbia; and Dr. Josée Lavoie, professor in Community Health Sciences, University of Manitoba, the BSWG was formed in response to Sinclair's death and the questions it raised for health care, the justice system, Indigenous people, and the province of Manitoba.[1] This coming together of people to form a critical discussion group is nothing new in terms of Indigenous and allied activism in Winnipeg. We saw it in the response of the Manitoba Indian Brotherhood to the 1969 White Paper; we see it today in the founding and return of the Bear Clan Patrol, in Meet Me at the Bell Tower, and in Friends of Shoal Lake 40.[2]

Such groups of committed, engaged individuals have offered valuable professional and grassroots insights into critical issues affecting life in Winnipeg and beyond, and the BSWG is similar. We do this work to record and analyze pressing issues, to raise awareness and promote equity, and to act in ways that foster change and create a public consciousness that includes Indigenous communities. In the fall of 2017, the BSWG released a fifteen-page report, *Out of Sight*, which contains the BSWG's interim recommendations, along with a summary of the events leading up to Brian Sinclair's death and the institutional responses to it.[3] The work of the BSWG constitutes a valuable archive of the lived immediacy of colonization and resistance in the everyday, ordinary present. The work of the BSWG and other resources are compiled on the "For Brian Sinclair" webpage created and maintained by BSWG member and University of Manitoba librarian Janice Linton.[4]

Structures of Indifference aims to augment the work of the BSWG and locate Sinclair's life and death within the overlapping histories of Winnipeg, Manitoba, and Canadian hospitals and health care, particularly health care and services for Indigenous people. In putting Sinclair's story in historical context, we draw on our collective expertise as historians; in McCallum's case, of Indigenous people, health care, and gender in twentieth-century Canada; in Perry's, of colonialism and western Canada in the nineteenth and twentieth centuries. Our primary archive is the substantial one created by the inquest that examined Sinclair's death. The inquest was held in Winnipeg in two phases: the first, in August and October of 2013, ran for thirty-two days and heard evidence from seventy-four witnesses. The second phase was shorter and more limited in scope. Early in the second phase, Brian Sinclair's family members and two important Indigenous organizations (Aboriginal Legal Services, a Toronto-based legal advocacy organization, and Ka Ni Kanichihk, a Winnipeg organization that offers culturally based and Indigenous-led social services) withdrew, having lost confidence in the inquest process. The second phase of the inquest met in January and February of 2014, and heard from ten witnesses.[5] The transcript of testimony to both phases of the inquest totals 4,653 pages. Manitoba Courts released a 200-page report on the inquest in December of 2014.[6] That this material is available online is largely owing to the fact that the Sinclair family, early in the inquest, petitioned the court to have the transcripts made public and free of cost.[7]

These materials produced through and around Sinclair's death are a particular kind of archive. Scholars of colonialism have argued that we need to be mindful of the shape of and work done by the records of colonial states. Ann Laura Stoler argues that we should pay attention "not only to colonialism's archival content, but to its particular and sometimes peculiar form," and view colonial archives "as both transparencies on which power relations were inscribed and intricate technologies of rule in themselves." Our social historians' training in reading against the grain, or from below, does not serve us well here. Instead, Stoler urges us to read *along* the archival grain, to attend to what the colonial archive offers and the multiple kinds of work that it does.[8] For example, the records of the inquest into Brian Sinclair's death are a window into a particular legal process defined in Canadian law. This process is not designed to illuminate the broader historical and colonial context in which events take place; rather the context is narrowly defined to make blanket recommendations on issues related to the inquest's interpretation of the event itself. As such, this archive reflects the precarious position of Indigenous people with respect to Canadian health care and justice, and how problematic this is for the care with which cases involving untimely deaths of Indigenous people are handled. Like Sherene Razack, we find that the inquest served to obscure the violence of colonialism; however, we wish to push this argument further by more precisely locating the inquest in specific histories of Indigenous people in Winnipeg and in Canadian hospitals.

The specific mode of colonialism practised in modern Canada is settler colonialism. Settler colonialism is sometimes defined as a form of colonialism where settlers came to stay, but that is too simple a definition. Mohawk scholar Audra Simpson explains that settler colonialism is at once an analytic, a social formation, an attitude, and an imaginary that helps us name "what happened and is still happening in spaces seized away from people, in ongoing projects to mask that seizure while attending to capital accumulation under another name."[9] Canadians are not used to this framing of their past as violent and ongoing. Until the last twenty-five years or so, Canadian history was mainly written as a benevolent, peaceful, and largely natural progression from a resource-rich hinterland to a modern multicultural state. Indigenous people in such renderings of history have a very little role— removed or erased from the land to facilitate settlement and resource extraction, they are "othered" by the newcomers who are the central protagonists in the story that is Canadian history.[10]

We think it is possible and indeed necessary to challenge this erasure of Indigenous people from Canadian history while recognizing the very real, persistent, and exhausting spectre of Indigenous death in Canadian cities. We are especially indebted to the work of Razack for our analysis of Sinclair's life and death and of the state mechanisms to examine, address, and archive them. Razack's generative scholarship on Indigenous deaths in custody in Canada offers a sharp and empirically grounded analysis of how settler colonialism's constituent and relentless logic works to render Indigenous people as already "always on the brink of death."[11] Her analysis is especially helpful in understanding the catastrophe of Sinclair's death, its aftermath, and the search to pin the cause of his death on his own person and actions in order to make sense of it. Razack argues that the energy that is expended to deny racism and colonialism is testimony to settlers' continuing need to obliterate a people; settlers cannot seamlessly or easily become the original citizens if Indigenous people remain and thrive.

Scholarship in Indigenous studies helps us see how these dynamics work on the ground in colonized spaces like Winnipeg. Here we draw on and aim to contribute to a range of conversations that address what we might call the Indigenous everyday. Everyday Indigenous experience exists in spite of efforts to remove and destroy Indigenous peoples, or, more casually, to ignore or singularly pathologize them. Histories of colonialism continue to revisit and frequently interrupt our ordinary lives, often in painful and jarring ways, for instance, when we are chairing a hiring committee, while we are having a cast put on a broken leg, while we innocently overhear or cannot silence the same old conversations that deny the violence of residential schools. We can register these moments as reminders that history is not over. We can also let them remind us of points made by Indigenous studies scholars Audra Simpson, Kim Tallbear, Beth Piatote, Philip J. Deloria, Brendan Hokowithu, Sarah Hunt, and others. In different ways, these scholars show how Indigenous humanity is powerfully asserted in everyday acts that illuminate colonial practices, challenge generalizations, and renew an ongoing presence in and relationship to where Indigenous people live. Here we locate local indigeneity within this everyday and ordinary experience of Winnipeg and we seek ways to see the city, the hospital, and Brian Sinclair's life and death in this way.

We also rely on settler colonial studies. Settler historian of Australia Patrick Wolfe offers us the critical observation that settler colonialism must be understood as a structure, not an event; as ongoing and diffuse rather than historical and contained.[12]

This observation recognizes that acquiring Indigenous lands "can be accomplished in overt ways including biological warfare and military domination but also in more subtle ways; for example, through national policies of assimilation."[13] The conquest of Indigenous territories does not just happen through guns, diseases, and administrative systems. It also happens through ideas and ideologies—including ideas about race and ideas about what counts as racism in a state that sees itself as "new," as "democratic," and as "free." Razack argues, however, that here in Canada, the dominant ideology of settler colonialism consigns Indigenous peoples "forever to an earlier space and time" and positions people of colour as terminal "late arrivals," assigning both agency and innocence to European settlers.[14] The Indian Act anchored Indigenous–state relations in the nineteenth century, rendering First Nations populations subject to a separate system of Canadian law and to legal definitions developed especially for First Nations people and without their input. Amended regularly but only ever partially, the Indian Act defines Indian people, resources, and land and determines how they will be managed and to what end; it also defines a set of laws and governing structures that reflect those objectives. This separate system filters throughout many aspects of law, including health and the development of Canadian health care systems. These systems, too, are ideologically driven structures of settler colonialism that draw on and in turn create ideas about race and indigeneity that reinforce claims of European settler populations as those first and most rightfully served by the state.

We also need to be mindful that Wolfe's framing can be read or used in ways that fail to recognize the lived history of settler colonialism in places like Winnipeg and double down on the erasure of Indigenous people. For example, by centring "the colonial" in our stories, it is sometimes difficult to see the very common and proportionally significant everyday lives of Indigenous people in the shared spaces in which we live. On this point, we take the intervention of Kanaka Maoli scholar Kēhaulani Kauanui, who reminds us that any analyses of settler colonialism must account for enduring indigeneity; first, that "Indigenous people exist, resist and persist; and second, that settler colonialism is a structure that endures indigeneity, as it holds out against it."[15] As historians, we are wary of analyses of the past that are built on a premise of Indigenous decline and that can replicate an endless colonial logic. In this book, we work to question and challenge the commonplace assumptions of Indigenous absence and write about how the settler colonial logic of erasure persists and works even where Indigenous people are very much present.

Like other western Canadian cities where Indigenous people form a significant and growing part of the population, Winnipeg conforms to, departs from, and complicates wider continental and global practices of understanding and framing Indigenous experience. A 2016 census identified 12.2 percent of Winnipeg's population as First Nations, Metis, or Inuit.[16] In this context, it is abundantly clear that for all the upheavals wrought by settler colonialism, Indigenous people remain in this space—real, unexceptional, and ordinary, and at times undeniably visible. The standard set of cultural tropes that shape the representation of Indigenous people in modern North America play out differently here. Historian Philip Deloria has written about "Indians in unexpected places," persisting when presumed absent. Jean O'Brien has analyzed the way that discourses of Indigenous disappearance—of the "first" settler and the "last" Indian—structure the way we minimize Indigenous historical experience.

These continental discourses and histories are part of the ones we describe here, though the weight of local histories and presents adds specificity and demands attention to particular dynamics of place and time.[17] Brian Sinclair was far from a singular or unusual Indigenous person in the HSC emergency ward, or downtown Winnipeg, on his last night in 2008. Sinclair was one man within a large and regular Indigenous presence in these spaces, and we must look beyond analyses that presume the rarity of the Indigenous person within settler colonial spaces to understand what happened to him and what we might learn from it.[18] Legal scholar Kimberlé Crenshaw's framing of intersectionality helps us here. Crenshaw argues that experiences like violence are shaped by the intersection of race and gender[19] and that meaningful interventions must account for this. In Chapter 3, we argue that Brian Sinclair's situation during those thirty-four hours reflected his experience not simply as a visibly Indigenous person, but as a middle-aged, significantly and visibly disabled man, and that our analysis must attend to gender, ability, and age as well as to indigeneity.

Indigeneity is not race, ethnicity, or nationality, even while it encompasses all of these at different times and is also minimized and harmed by them. Often definitions of indigeneity focus on legal implications or on individual and group identification or identity. Indeed, who can and should identify as Indigenous is a battleground for many in North America, in part because of the longstanding role the state has taken in defining who is and who is not Indigenous, and in part also because this entails a special relationship and rights derived from nation-to-nation treaties with the federal government of Canada. While the state maintains a significant stake in defining indigeneity in Canada, as always, its practices in this regard are illusive, and we cannot rely on its registries of First Nations status people, for example, to define the meaning of Indigenous. Chris Andersen argues in his book *Metis: Race,*

Recognition, and the Struggle for Indigenous People-hood that racialization, blood, and concepts of racial mixedness and purity have come to define indigeneity in ways that diminish Indigenous peoplehood and history. He points to a concept of "Indigenous collective self-awareness" instead of state-recognized legal categories defined by others. In practice, being Indigenous means coming from or belonging to the land one inhabits and having a primary and historical connection to place and to one another.[20] At the same time, Indigenous people and indigeneity are socially constructed categories borne of the history of settler colonialism in settler colonial societies.

While indigeneity is not analogous to race, Indigenous people can and do experience racism, and thinking about systemic racism is critical to understanding histories of Indigenous people, including those of individuals like Sinclair. One effect of anti-Indigenous racism is what we call structures of indifference. The structures of indifference that Brian Sinclair encountered—where he was literally ignored to death—are on regular display throughout Canada. They are not simply a manifestation of individuals holding negative or bigoted views of Indigenous people and treating them poorly; racist acts are qualitatively diverse and pervasive. They are also more than bald statistics that point to the poorer health, shorter lifespans, and lack of basic necessities experienced by Indigenous people.

Racism influences people's lives in ways that simply cannot be reduced to statistics and bullet points.

This book is indebted to the work of Janet Smylie, Charlotte Reading, Yvonne Boyer, Margo Greenwood, Sarah De Leeuw, Annette Browne, and many others who have sought to describe anti-Indigenous racism in the Canadian context, identify race and racism as social determinants of health, locate particular sites of health inequity, and make policy recommendations.[21] We find that in its emphasis on intervention and future health change, Indigenous health research has a tendency to invoke history in narrow and instrumentalist ways and to inadvertently depict Indigenous health, health care, and research as distinct from and as successors to, rather than products of, settler colonial history. Work that identifies racism in health care tends to recommend generalized implicit bias and cultural safety training—primarily for health professionals, and most commonly physicians. While training programs are an important step, they tend to focus on Indigenous "culture" and not racism, and in so doing they implicitly re-centre and privilege whiteness as the normative perspective while failing to address the myriad ways that racism deprives people of opportunities and structures their lives. What is more, they often aim to identify and neutralize stereotypes or misconceptions about people with uncritical, dry, crude accounts of history.[22]

In this book, we bring some of the tools of history to contextualize racism in health care and, more specifically, Brian Sinclair's death and the inquest into it. We use generalized statistics, but we do so in ways that are grounded in critical Indigenous-centred and intersectional readings of specific contexts. We query the colonial frames of medicine and health that have produced Indigenous blood and bodies as special subjects of inquiry, intervention, and discipline and acknowledge them as structures that create and maintain inequities. We seek to understand racism not as a set of individually held beliefs or actions against a backdrop of history, but as a structure of indifference—one that shapes and produces life chances.[23] We seek to discern how structures support, enable, and inform putatively individual actions. And above all, we seek a more complicated, local analysis that is attentive to place and time. In the context of Winnipeg and Manitoba, and indeed Canada and other parts of the settler colonial world, oversimplified and nationalist histories must be understood for the role they play in the continuing practice of settler colonial structures. When we separate the history of people like Brian Sinclair and institutions like the HSC and cities like Winnipeg from the wider history of the dispossession of Indigenous people and land, we radically misunderstand and underestimate the context—the structures—that shape our lived experiences. We try to get beyond an unhelpful debate about whether it was individual or structural racism that killed Brian Sinclair. Rather, we insist that settler colonialism, and the structures of indifference that it produces and is maintained by, are always both.

Colonization involved a much broader social, cultural, and political agenda that involved the organization of special services and programs for Indigenous people, including in the area of health. Colonization has had a physical impact on the health of Indigenous people—most obviously in the devastation of Indigenous populations.[24] The colonial history of Indigenous health also involves the supplanting of Indigenous health and health care practices and the undermining of Indigenous knowledge related to health. The imposition of a limited and understaffed separate system of Indian Health Services in the twentieth century ensured that, while the health of Indigenous people declined and Indigenous health knowledge was being replaced, further colonization was justified, sustained; even applauded.[25]

In Canada, our investment in racism is such that it serves to ensure the state and settlers' continued access to land and a claim to sovereignty over it. That is, racism in Canada is tied to a historically rooted but also continuing practice of claiming and organizing Indigenous land and people. To acknowledge Indigenous people as equals in Canada would be to acknowledge the validity of Indigenous claims to territory and self-governance. It would also mean acknowledging that race—and more specifically white supremacy—is profoundly embedded in the ways in which our systems operate. A desire to mould Canada into a distinctly white settler state is evident, for example, in the dispossession, removal, and discipline of Indigenous people; the exclusion, segregation, and marginalization of people of colour; and the creation and repetition of pervasive national narratives about Canada that valorize white settlement and governance.

Yet we understand racism also to be specific to time, place, and context. In the medical field, racist practices are embedded in a long and nationwide history of racial segregation in hospitals, and notions of who is and who is not deserving of medical care and what that care might look like are intimately tied to political, economic, religious, technological, and cultural influences. The many ways in which racism is embedded in Canadian history, however, also show how, over time, cultural narratives can and do change, because history, and how we tell and understand it, is not static. There is indeed potential for change, which is why it is important to discuss longstanding systemic issues of racism in Canada.

Thinking about settler colonialism and intersectionality allows us to complicate an analysis of racism in spaces that may look desegregated and progressive, and maybe even Indigenous, and to see some of the ways in which Indigenous people experience cities like Winnipeg. To discuss Brian Sinclair's last thirty-four hours and the inquest that documented them is to engage directly with a painful, difficult, and traumatic history. People who have had a traumatic experience at a hospital—or have been with a loved one who they felt was not being properly cared for—may feel this history. People who have felt at some point that they are being discriminated against in institutions that purport to help might feel this especially, as in the case of Indigenous and racialized people. In presenting this work to different audiences, we have learned that it affects people deeply and that it is important to notify audiences of this; we provide a list of some local resources below.* In reflecting on trauma and history writing, we find the work of Metis scholars Jesse Thistle and Zoe Todd helpful. Thistle writes about the trauma of historical research into stories of loss and dispossession, of the ways that his "ancestor's stories linger and revisit . . . and harm [him] as they are trying to be remembered."[26] There can be—and often are—corrosive

---

* Readers who find the histories discussed here traumatic can consider contacting the resources made available through the First Nations and Inuit Hope for Wellness Help Line at 1-855-242-3310, the Indian Residential Schools Resolution Health Support Program at 1-866-925-4419, or, in Winnipeg, the Klinic Community Health Centre's 24-Hour Crisis Line at 1-888-322-3019.

relationships and impacts when Indigenous trauma is relayed, especially by non-Indigenous scholars and writers. Zoe Todd reminds readers that non-Indigenous scholars can walk away from lived traumas that define Indigenous lives, and that Indigenous historical trauma has become a form of capital for settler scholars while colonial violence experienced by Indigenous people is ongoing.[27]

As authors and scholars, we draw on our experiences as a Lenape historian from Ontario (McCallum) and as a non-Indigenous scholar and historian from British Columbia (Perry). In this book we aim to be mindful of the limits on what we know and responsibly tell. We have both spent the substantial part of our working lives in Winnipeg, and this book is very much written from here. We try to capture the details of how colonialism is lived on this ground. In the Conclusion, we return to some of the ways this has been driven home in the last year, but these details are also embedded in legal processes that routinely deny racism, the commonplace framing of Indigenous ill-health as in part an effort to erase people who refuse to be erased, and the fact that unnatural Indigenous deaths in health-care settings and elsewhere occur frequently. The records we draw on are public and easily available online, and this project has been undertaken with the permission of Brian Sinclair's family. In honour of Sinclair and his relatives, we have directed the University of Manitoba Press to send royalties from the sale of this book to Ka Ni Kanichihk, an Indigenous-run service organization in Winnipeg that played an important role in the effort to demand a rigorous response to Sinclair's death.[28]

As McCallum has argued elsewhere, we need to frame our recognition of trauma in an understanding that Indigenous history was and is much more than a story of loss; multiple forms of experience can and do coexist.[29] We also need to hold in balance our concern with the politics and ethics of rehashing, and the inherent risk of reinflicting, Indigenous trauma with the need to engage with these difficult histories that surround us. The story of Brian Sinclair's life and death is one of an Indigenous man who was continually ignored in a space specifically designated to provide care. It tells us a great deal about the city of Winnipeg, the province, and the country in which this tragedy occurred, and the structures of indifference made and remade in and through our colonial past and present.

The Health Sciences Centre Security Services' direct video recording left a powerful visual archive of Brian Sinclair's last thirty-four hours. In a way, the impersonal recordings represent the only entity that consistently "saw" Brian Sinclair, and thus the video footage is an important witness. We begin with those thirty-four hours and that archive before proceeding to three chapters that document different sites and the histories in and around them: the city, the hospital, and Sinclair himself.

TIMELINE[30]

Brian Sinclair arrived at the Health Sciences Centre Emergency Department at 2:53 p.m. on Friday, 19 September. He was experiencing pain and needed assistance with the catheter bag he used. He had already been to the Health Action Centre, a community clinic and his usual health care provider, where he had been seen first by a nurse and then by a family physician. They determined that his catheter needed to be changed and that he should go to the HSC's emergency department for this procedure, because they wanted the catheter change the be done in a sterile environment, they were not sure they could lift him, and they wanted him to be able to obtain quick results from the necessary lab tests. Because his condition was stable, the physician told Sinclair that she would arrange transportation. At first, Sinclair offered to wheel himself to the ER, but staff arranged for a taxi. Before he left, Brian Sinclair was given a letter about his condition and was told to give the letter to a nurse at the HSC.

As seen in the video footage, when Sinclair arrived at the HSC, he was alert and wheeled himself to the triage desk. He was greeted by a triage aide, seen on the video interacting with Sinclair for about thirty seconds. The aide's job was to record Sinclair's name, time of arrival, and medical issue. While the aide later testified that he did not recall if he had, the inquest determined that "he appeared to have done none of these things.... He did not keep track of Brian Sinclair."[31] As a result, Sinclair was not recorded as a patient who needed to be assessed by the triage nurse. Security camera footage shows that Sinclair undertook the same steps entering the ER as patients who arrived after him, all of whom "were triaged and assessed by Triage Nurses."[32]

After his brief interaction with the aide, Sinclair wheeled himself into a corner behind the security desk. He took the letter from his physician out of his pocket and then put it away a short while later. For the whole time he was in the HSC ER, Sinclair was positioned in a way that he was visible to people walking around the ER.

Brian Sinclair had several interactions over the next thirty-four hours. At 3:15 p.m., the security camera recorded Sinclair moving in front of the security desk, wheeling himself past the triage desk area, and then wheeling himself to park his wheelchair near the security desk. At 3:37 p.m., Sinclair can be seen returning from the washroom area of the waiting room. At about 3:40 p.m., Sinclair was asked by a security guard to move from the security desk area, and he did so. At about 6:00 p.m., he wheeled himself to the security desk and spoke with a guard. The video shows that by 8:01 p.m. he was slumped in his wheelchair, where he remained until the early morning of the next day.

A nurse checked on patients in the waiting room in the early morning hours of Saturday, 20 September. This nurse knew Sinclair by name, and at some point between 3:00 a.m. and 5:00 a.m. she spoke to him. His response was garbled, and in her inquest testimony she described him as lethargic, but she did not ask Sinclair how he was feeling or determine whether he had seen a doctor.

At 3:41 a.m., Sinclair wheeled himself back into the waiting room from the washroom area, and the video shows him slumped in his chair again. At approximately 4:00 a.m., a triage nurse moved through the waiting room, checking on the status of people there who had been triaged and were waiting to see a physician. He testified that he checked Brian Sinclair's wrist to see if he was wearing a wristband, which would indicate that he had been triaged. Because Sinclair was sleeping and was not wearing a wristband, the triage nurse assumed either that Sinclair had been discharged earlier and was waiting for a pickup or that he was homeless and seeking shelter, or that he had been brought in and detained under the Intoxicated Persons Detention Act. In any event, the triage nurse did not speak to Sinclair and made no further inquiries. At 4:39 a.m., Sinclair can again be seen on the video wheeling himself out of the washroom area. For the rest of Saturday morning, he sat in his wheelchair, the video camera capturing his movements and shifts in body position.

In the early afternoon, Sinclair vomited. A man whose son was a patient in the emergency waiting room said he noticed Brian Sinclair right away because he looked obviously distressed. At 12:42 p.m. that day, the man approached the nearby security guard and told him that a man was vomiting. The guard called housekeeping to clean up the vomit but did not alert medical staff. He saw that Sinclair was motionless and had his eyes closed but assumed he was intoxicated and "sleeping it off." He testified that he made this assumption because "Sinclair looked to him like someone who was intoxicated."[33]

Later in the afternoon, the same man in the waiting room again saw Brian Sinclair vomit and again alerted the security guard because he thought Sinclair needed help. While housekeeping staff cleaned up and provided a basin, no health care staff responded to Sinclair's vomiting or to the request for help from a member of the public.

On the afternoon of 20 September, a nurse practitioner saw Sinclair and noticed the basin he had been given after he vomited. She took this as a sign that someone else had attended to him and did not check if he needed care. Later in the day, she passed Brian Sinclair, whose head was slumped to the side. She assumed that he was sleeping, that someone had already taken care of him, and that he was just wait-ing for a bed in another area.

On Saturday evening, a couple waiting in the emergency room with their daughter also intervened on behalf of Sinclair. They had first come to the HSC on the evening of Friday, 19 September, and when they returned the following evening, the woman was alarmed because she noticed that Sinclair was still in the same position. She approached a student nurse and explained her concern. The student nurse replied that people stay in the waiting room after they are released because they have nowhere else to go and that homeless people use the ER to sleep and stay warm. The woman also told a security supervi-sor that she thought someone should check on him, but no one did. The final video image of Sinclair, captured at 11:45 p.m. that night, shows him in the same location he was in at 4:37 p.m. the previous day.

21 SEPTEMBER 2008

Just after midnight, the same woman again ap-proached a security guard because she was concerned that Sinclair had not moved and she feared he was dead. At first, the guard replied that he was probably just intoxicated, but when she insisted that something was wrong, the guard went over to Sinclair. When he did not respond to being tapped and pinched, the guard realized Sinclair was dead and wheeled him to nursing staff. Medical personnel attempted CPR, but

Brian Sinclair was pronounced dead at 12:51 a.m. on 21 September 2008. The doctor's letter that he was to give to a nurse was found in his jacket pocket.

By the time Sinclair's death was discovered, rigor mortis had set in and a precise time of death could not be established; however, it had been "at least hours."[34] The cause of death was acute peritonitis that was a consequence of severe acute cystitis, or inflammation of the bladder. The severe infection (sepsis) Sinclair experienced caused his abdominal cavity to become inflamed and his blood pressure to drop. There was inadequate blood flow to the vital organs, including his brain, which led to a loss of consciousness and hypotensive shock. The autopsy confirmed that he did not have drugs or alcohol in his system. Sinclair's family said he was simply "ignored to death."[35]

The HSC ER is the most comprehensive medical facility serving Manitoba and northwestern Ontario. There were 150 other people who came to the ER between the time of Sinclair's arrival, 2:53 p.m. on Friday, 19 September, and the time that he was declared dead at 12:51 a.m. on Sunday, 21 September. They were all triaged and either treated by a medical professional or left voluntarily without treatment.

Brian Sinclair came to the HSC ER seeking urgent but not critical care. He did not leave the ER. Had he received the care he needed, he would not have died. His presence in the waiting room was visible to HSC staff, but, again and again, he was not identified by hospital staff as a patient needing care. Rather, he was visible as an Indigenous man, not as a patient—despite being in a wheelchair, in an ER, with obvious signs of medical distress that were recognized by other patients. No staff members asked him why he was still in the waiting room at any point during the thirty-four hours that elapsed after he wheeled himself in because they assumed that he was homeless, intoxicated, or just hanging around. Even as his condition worsened, no medical personnel recognized him as a patient in distress. Even when members of the public intervened on his behalf, HSC ER staff members were quick to explain that Brian Sinclair was not ill but simply sleeping or intoxicated. This assumption, made and remade over and over in the thirty-four hours while Sinclair sickened and died in a hospital ER, is a striking and painful example of one of the structures of indifference that cost Brian Sinclair his life, as it has cost the lives of other Indigenous people in Canadian cities.

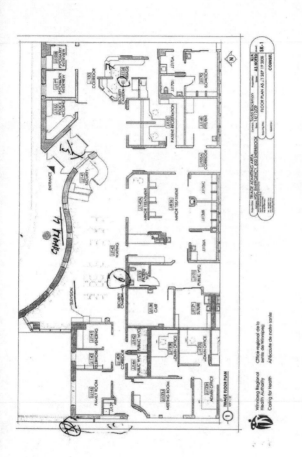

Figure 2. This map was marked up by Winnipeg Police Sergeant John O'Donovan. Assigned to the investigation into the death of Sinclair, O'Donovan had reviewed hundreds of hours of surveillance video, and his marks indicate the location from which each clip shown to the court was filmed. The map was entered into evidence at the inquest as Exhibit 15.

THE CITY

①

THE INDIGENOUS LIFE AND DEATH that this book discusses occurred within a particular city, province, and nation, and this context is the focus of this chapter. The histories of colonialism and dispossession we engage here are pervasive and global. But they are also local and specific. To understand what happened to Brian Sinclair during those thirty-four hours in 2008, we need to begin with the particular place in which it occurred. This approach helps bring to light the intricacies of the colonial project and how it produced the death of Brian Sinclair. In offering a place-based historical account, we illustrate the enduring presence of Indigenous people here. We begin with the city of Winnipeg and the province of Manitoba within the nation state of Canada.

The city where Brian Sinclair lived most of his life and spent his last thirty-four hours is located on the storied and ancient lands of Anishinaabeg, Cree, and Metis people. The Red and Assiniboine Rivers connected Anishinaabeg and Cree communities to

Indigenous people throughout the Americas. Archaeological research confirms oral archives that situate the Forks of the Red and Assiniboine Rivers as a site of human settlement and trade for at least 6,000 years.[1] Records indicating Indigenous agriculture at the Forks are confirmed by archaeological evidence of intensive agriculture dating from the early 1400s.[2] The inhabitants of these lands were not static societies awaiting European arrival, but societies in motion and transition. Anishinaabeg people came west from Lake of the Woods in the late eighteenth century and were welcomed through traditional protocols by Cree and Assiniboine people.[3]

These territories were part of the expansive space that was, in 1670, claimed, in an odd sort of imperial way, as both British and Hudson's Bay Company (HBC) territory. As historian Michael Witgen argues, "Laying claim to possession of the western interior in this fashion was, for all practical purposes, an action of political fiction."[4] Britain and its colonial settlements were a long distance away, and this expanse of land remained very much an Indigenous space occasionally interrupted by a small post defended by a few garrisoned soldiers. The arrival of a modest number of settlers in 1812 shifted but did not radically alter the fact that this remained an Indigenous place.

From the late eighteenth century onwards, the Forks of the Red and Assiniboine Rivers were a particular space of Metis community. The Metis

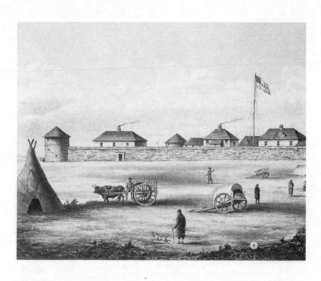

Figure 3. A nostalgic vision of Upper Fort Garry, built in 1822 near the forks of the Red and Assiniboine Rivers. This was painted around 1881, about the time when the fort was demolished.

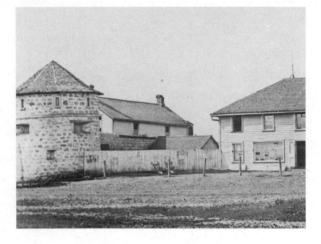

Figure 4. Upper Fort Garry in the 1870s.
Located in what is now downtown Winnipeg,
the fort was the site of the meeting of the
Legislative Assembly of Assiniboia under the
leadership of Louis Riel in the summer of
1870, and where Wolseley's troops were
later garrisoned.

are a post-contact Indigenous people anchored in land, culture, and history.[5] Particularly critical here was a series of interconnected communities along the lengths of both rivers known by a number of names, but most often as the Red River colony or settlement. By the middle decades of the nineteenth century, Red River was a thriving and overwhelmingly Metis society. Of the roughly 12,000 people enumerated as permanent residents in Red River in 1870, about 10,000 were described as either "half-breed" or "Metis," and another 560 as "settled Indians" with homes and farms. Of the 1,563 who were enumerated as "white," nearly half had been born in the Northwest and were likely to have had lineage and kin ties that linked them, in a variety of ways, to Indigenous people.[6]

Historian Damon Salesa has shown how nineteenth-century racial logic was both global and remarkably local.[7] On the one hand, racial thinking and practice were consolidated and instrumentalized in the middle years of the nineteenth century. Yet this process played out in particular ways, including in the fur trade and in and around Red River. Intimate relationships and families formed by white men and Indigenous women that had been the bedrock of fur-trade society became less common, especially for the elite. A series of high-profile controversies in Red River worked to cumulatively undermine the moral authority of Indigenous women. In the eighteenth and early nineteenth centuries Indigenous men regularly rose in the colonial and fur-trade ranks if they had sufficient family resources, connections, and skills.[8] This changed, in large part if not entirely, in the years following the reorganization of the western fur trade in 1821. By the 1830s, it was rare for Indigenous men to be promoted beyond the rank of postmaster.[9]

Yet Red River's powerful Indigenous elite survived these challenges of the 1820s and 1830s. Alexander Kennedy Isbister (1803–1890) was born to a Cree-Metis mother and an Orcadian father. Isbister excelled at school in Red River, but when he joined the HBC service he was predictably, and insultingly, appointed to the position of postmaster. Isbister left Red River for the United Kingdom, where he trained as a barrister and moved in influential, upwardly mobile circles. In correspondence he endeavoured to explain the particular, layered colonial society of his homeland, and its Indigenous elite, to a confused British public. In 1859, Isbister explained that, "with the exception of the small Scotch community at Red River and a few missionaries' wives, every married woman and mother of a family above the grade of an Indian throughout the whole extent of the Hudson's Bay Territories, is of mixed race, and is with her children the inheritor of all the wealth of the country—the fortunes made in the fur-trade, and the valuable property accumulated in the Red River Colony—must of itself invest this class with a high degree of interest and importance." The sons of HBC officers, he went on, had inherited "often considerable property," were "generally well educated (many of them in universities in Great Britain, Canada and the United States)," and occupied the usual positions of the local elite, including "the Sheriff of the Red River Colony, the medical officers, the surveyors, the postmaster, the entire staff of the teachers in schools and a fair proportion of the Clergy of the Christian Missionaries and other societies," as well as the "Municipal Council of the Red River Settlement."[10]

The last third of the nineteenth century was a complicated and consequential time for this part of the world. A series of linked colonial manoeuvres variously occurred in London and Ottawa via some important legislation: first, the British North America Act (1867), which created Canada as a particular sort of nation within the British Empire, one with distinct imperial ambitions of its own with respect to the territories lying to its north and west; second, Britain's Rupertsland Act in 1868; and third, Canada's 1869 "Act for the Temporary Government of Rupert's Land." As Adam Gaudry explains, these three pieces of legislation were thought to "unilaterally transfer the possession of a vast peopled landscape from one authority of empire, the Hudson's Bay Company, to another—Canada."[11] Under the leadership of Louis Riel, Red River would object, strenuously, militarily, and successfully, to these acts of colonial fiat and establish their own government. The winter of 1869–70 was a tumultuous one, including the execution of Canadian Thomas Scott by the provisional government for refusing to acknowledge its authority.

As a direct result of this resistance, Manitoba entered Confederation not as a colony of Canada, but as a small province within it, set by the terms of the Manitoba Act of 1870. Manitoba was the only Canadian province to enter Confederation on its own, explicitly Metis, terms, and in armed conflict. The early months of Manitoba's existence as a province suggested that this history and these aspirations would persist: in the summer of 1870, electors, including "settled Indians" from St. Peter's, and maybe even some women, elected the Legislative Assembly of Assiniboia. Twenty-one of its twenty-eight members were Metis, half French- or Michif-speaking and half English-speaking; most also spoke Cree or Anishnaabemowin.[12] What would unfold over the next few decades, however, would create a city and a province that looked very different from what people at Red River may have imagined in the 1860s, and fought for during the long winter of 1869–70.

The transformation of Red River from this layered, variegated Indigenous place into a Canadian and settler space was accomplished in a number of ways, including sustained violence. Historians of Red River refer to a "reign of terror" between 1870 and

1872. The Red River Expeditionary Force, made up of more than 1,000 Canadian militiamen, arrived in 1870 and was garrisoned at Upper Fort Garry, in what became a nest of buildings representing the new colonial order, and which included the Dominion Lands Office. The force was led by Colonel Garnet Wolseley, whose imperial military career was built on the suppression of rebellion and on the seizure of land and assets across the globe, in Burma, Crimea, India, and, after Red River, Africa.[13] The soldiers have been described as poorly disciplined, but Wolseley was an experienced military man, and we can see that his troops worked to actively displace the local elite. The year before he arrived in Red River, Wolseley published *Soldiers' Pocket Book for Field Service*, which "enter[ed] into the most minute details on everything connected with the wild life one has to lead in the field, when cut adrift, perhaps, entirely from civilisation."[14] Riel and A.D. Lepine attested that "the conduct of Wolseley was a real calamity. It produced its victims."[15] Metis newspapers came under attack, as did the electoral process and the community's leadership.[16] Riel was elected to the Parliament of Canada for Provencher, Manitoba, in both 1873 and 1874, but owing to backlash in Ottawa he was never able to take his seat.[17] The list of Metis men beaten or killed in these years is chilling: François Guillemette was killed on the trail one night; André Nault was beaten nearly to death; Elzéar Goulet drowned fleeing a gang that included the father-in-law of the governor; Joseph Dubuc, a lawyer and member of the new provincial legislature, was beaten and left blind in one eye; Curtis Bird, Speaker of the Legislative Assembly, was tarred—a public and physically dangerous form of ritualistic shaming in the late nineteenth century—for his opposition to a bill that would have incorporated Winnipeg in 1873. Bird "never really recovered."[18]

The attacks on Metis people and institutions in the 1870s were instrumental to the dispossession of the Metis from the region that was being remade as Winnipeg. Metis historian Fred J. Shore argues that mob violence at a critical time made it difficult for Metis to retain a foothold in the administration of the new province. In 1870, about half of the members of the Manitoba Legislature were Metis; nine years later, only four out of twenty-four were.[19] And there was the matter of land, the particular terrain of contest and struggle in settler colonial societies. Section 31 of the Manitoba Act promised 1.4 million acres to the children of "half-breed" heads of families residing in the province; section 32 guaranteed land tenure predating July 1870; section 32.5 guaranteed hay and common rights to Metis heads of families; additional legislation in 1874 granted Metis heads of families each $160 in scrip, redeemable in Dominion lands. For all the debate about Metis lands in Manitoba after 1870, there is no real debate about the loss of land: "very little of this land and

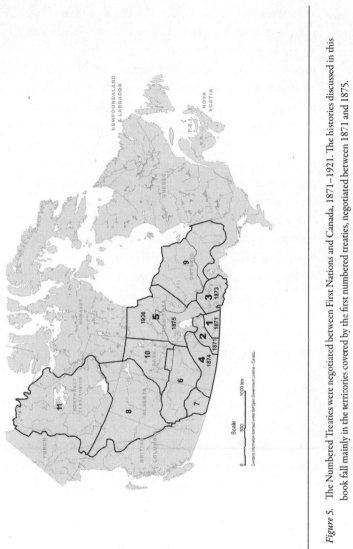

Figure 5. The Numbered Treaties were negotiated between First Nations and Canada, 1871–1921. The histories discussed in this book fall mainly in the territories covered by the first numbered treaties, negotiated between 1871 and 1875.

scrip remained in Metis hands by the late 1870s."[20] A toxic combination of fraud, confusion, speculation, and policy favouring incoming settlers from the east meant that Metis lands were taken over by newcomers. Many Metis, maybe as much as two-thirds of the population, moved west and north, where they had kin and (if briefly) land and economic opportunity.[21]

At the same time, First Nations were moving to permanent settlements on lands outside the city as demarcated in treaties. There had been a long Indigenous history of treaty-making in connection to this area where the Red and Assiniboine Rivers meet. Europeans entered into Indigenous practices of diplomacy, as with the Selkirk or Peguis Treaty of 1817. Marked by Anishinaabeg dodems, this treaty allowed for non-Indigenous settlement in specific quarters and arranged for annual payments. Most of all, it established ongoing relationships.[22] It was superseded by Treaty 1, the first of the "numbered treaties" negotiated between Canada and First Nations from Lake of the Woods to the Rocky Mountains, between 1871 and 1921 (see Figure 5). These treaties represented the reality of Canada's settler state power and both the possibilities and the limits of First Nations' capacity to resist and negotiate. But Indigenous and local histories of treaty-making remained. Locally, Treaty 1 was known as the Stone Fort Treaty, referring to the old fort of Lower Fort Garry, the site of nine days of treaty negotiations in the summer of 1871.

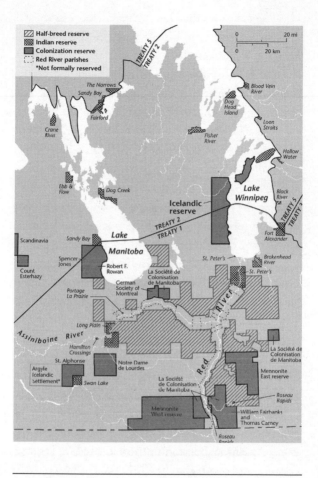

Figure 6. Map of reserves and surveyed lands in Manitoba, 1875. In the 1870s, what gradually became Manitoba was multiply divided into "reserves" for different groups of Indigenous people and European migrants.

The surname that Brian Sinclair bore associates him with these long histories of the fur trade and Metis in and around the Forks of the Red and Assiniboine. Manitoba Metis history is full of Sinclairs, one of a cluster of surnames—including Inkster, Tait, and Norquay—that give enduring evidence of ties between the Orkney Islands, the fur trade, and a Metis society rooted at Red River.[23] Sinclair's family history also tied him to First Nations in Manitoba, most notably the Anishinaabeg communities of Fort Alexander and Berens River, and with them, to the history of the numbered treaties and the legal and political histories of First Nations and the Canadian state.

The histories of many Indigenous families span both Metis and First Nations identities and experiences. In different ways, the research of Heather Devine on the Dejarlais family and of Robert Alexander Innes on kinship in and around Cowessess First Nation in Saskatchewan illustrates the points where Metis and plains First Nations were tied by kinship and proximity.[24] Brian Sinclair's specific lineage tied him to Fort Alexander, or Sagkeeng First Nation, an Anishinaabeg nation in Treaty 1, and to Berens River, an Anishinaabeg community located in Treaty 5. Treaty 1 was completed in 1871 and Treaty 5 in 1876, both part of the first wave of numbered treaties. The text of these treaties was similar, written in prose that adopted Indigenous reckonings of kinship and relationship, promising that First Nations "cede, release, yield up and surrender" land in exchange for modest annuities and reserved lands. First Nations' archives, including oral ones, speak of additional promises not recorded in the official versions preserved in colonial archives, and, profoundly, of a different meaning of treaty. "Indigenous people have their own views about treaties," explains Aimée Craft, asserting that they were indeed promises to share the land and resources, not give them up.[25]

The Manitoba Act and Treaties 1 through 5 signalled the remaking of Manitoba by the government of Canada. They coincided with developments in immigration policy and practice, including Canada's efforts to resettle prairie lands with non-Indigenous people through the 1872 Dominion Lands Act and the "block" settlement of Icelanders and German-speaking Mennonites from Russia. Historian Ryan Eyford shows us that the net result of these twinned processes of dispossession and colonization was a landscape remade, much of it divided into parcels of land "reserved" for one group or another, as shown in Figure 6.[26]

At the centre of this remade imperial space was Winnipeg, incorporated as a city in 1874 after a failed attempt in 1873, a tangible symbol of a new order finding its institutional footing. Older patterns of population persisted for another two decades, and Winnipeg for much of the 1870s and 1880s looked much like Red River. "The streets at all hours of the day present a curious mixture of civilization and savagery," opined one Canadian visitor.[27] Feminist author Nellie McClung recalled arriving in Winnipeg in 1880 as a child. Her reminiscences of her early days on the edges of what was becoming Winnipeg tell us a lot about Indigenous persistence, and how it could be seen as a threat to settler opportunity, including that of McClung's family, recently arrived from Ontario. McClung played with and liked "Indian Tommy," whose mother worked for hers. McClung's Ontario family decided not to buy "Louis Pruden's farm on the riverbank," since her mother found the place too Indigenous. "'Let us go on,' she said. 'Let us go to an all-white settlement. There are too many jet black eyes and high cheek bones here.'"[28]

But the loss of land and political power that occurred throughout the 1870s laid the groundwork for enduring demographic changes in the 1880s, 1890s, and especially the early 1900s. With the completion of the transcontinental railroad in 1885 and shifts in immigration practice and policy after 1896, Winnipeg's population began to change. In the early decades of the twentieth century it grew, and grew dramatically: in 1902, the city recorded a population of a little under 45,000; four years later, it was over 100,000.[29] This was a place remade, not just through the redrawing of maps and strokes of politicians' pens, but through the aspirations of people who saw the territories west of the Great Lakes as a space for imperial and colonial improvement, through technologies—including the railways—that made that more possible, and through the persistent movement of peoples, families, and lives across lakes and oceans. As historian Kurt Korneski explains, Winnipeg "emerged as a part of a nationalist project of settler colonialism."[30]

Early twentieth-century Winnipeg was a relentlessly ambitious and often bombastic place, the seat of a powerful cluster of capitalist and imperialist ambitions summed up in such aspirational phrases about the city as the "Gateway to the West" or the "Chicago of the North." As the Winnipeg General Strike of 1919 made clear, the city was also a locus for alternative visions of North America. Indigenous people were notably absent from this contest over Winnipeg's identity. Capitalists boasted of Winnipeg's industrial potential and labour radicals argued for a society based on human needs, not profits, but Indigenous people were rarely included in the discussion. To some extent, this erasure reflected the fact that the size of Winnipeg's Indigenous population reached all-time lows in the first two-thirds of the twentieth century, lower both than had been the case in the nineteenth century and than would become the case by the end of the twentieth century. In the first half of the twentieth century, explains geographer Evelyn Peters, Canada had expanded in a "largely segregated pattern of settlement."[31] From the 1880s onwards, federal policies, most notably

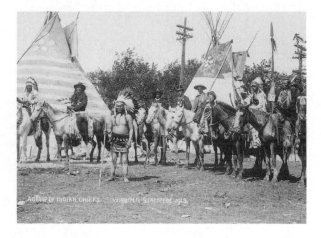

Figure 7.   As Indigenous people were made unwelcome in cities like Winnipeg and First Nations' ceremonies were outlawed, certain aspects of Indigenous cultures were put on display on city streets. Here is a "group of Indian Chiefs" at the Winnipeg Stampede in 1913.

the introduction of the Indian Act and the establishment of Indian residential schools, ordained that First Nations were very likely to live on reserves and, within the southern "settlement belt" of the prairies, were to be subject to a pass system, requiring permissions from an Indian agent to leave the reserve. A suite of semi-formal and informal policies worked to effectively shrink the geography of Indigenous lives and make cities such as Winnipeg at best unfriendly and at worst hostile places for Indigenous people. Historian Sarah Carter explains that "the disparities between the way most non-Aboriginal and Aboriginal Westerners lived and worked increased dramatically" from the mid-1890s onwards.[32]

Indigenous people who remained within Winnipeg did so in small numbers and under circumstances that were difficult or complicated, and often both. The census is likely to have underestimated the numbers of Indigenous people in the city, but even that measure recorded a small and persistent Indigenous population in the early part of the twentieth century. Between 1881 and 1916, between 0.3 percent and 1.6 percent of Winnipeg was described as Indian or Metis.[33] These figures did not include the municipalities, such as St. Boniface and St. Vital, that we might expect to have had significant Metis populations, even after the dispossession of many Metis families in the 1880s and 1890s. Urban Metis communities like Rooster Town hovered on the edges of Winnipeg's formal and informal boundaries.[34] The continuing presence of urban and suburban Indigenous people in Winnipeg occasioned anxiety from non-Indigenous people, and Indigenous people were thus subject to a range of extraordinary regulations. A study of early policing in Winnipeg indicates that police spent much of their time and resources monitoring First Nations and Metis people in the city and that "half-breed" was the most common "nationality" listed for people arrested in 1879 and 1880.[35]

These patterns would both persist and shift in the years following the Second World War. Indigenous populations everywhere were growing: the status Indian population of Manitoba grew 70.37 percent in the twenty-four years between 1934 and 1958.[36] The geography of segregation that had worked to ensure that "almost all" First Nations people lived on reserves from about 1900 onward began to break down in the 1950s.[37] Geographer Owen Toews identifies the cluster of changes that lay behind this movement to the city: the abolition of the pass system, ongoing dispossession of Indigenous lands and economies, faltering labour demand in northern resource industries, and the Department of Indian Affairs beginning to support certain kinds of urban migration.[38]

It was in these latter decades of the twentieth century that Winnipeg would begin what was in effect a process of re-Indigenization. The path travelled by Brian Sinclair's family, from both reserve and non-reserve Indigenous communities in Manitoba to the city of Winnipeg in the decades following the Second World War, was part of a wider history that was routinely registered in the local press. "Indians into Towns, Cities," proclaimed an article on the front page of the *Winnipeg Free Press* in 1958 (see Figure 8).[39] Non-governmental organizations and the Department of Indian Affairs both recorded steady rises in the urban First Nations population in Canada as a whole, and in Winnipeg in particular. In 1951, the Department of Indian Affairs reported 210 status Indians in the city; in 1961, 1,082; in 1971, 4,940; and in 1981, 16,757.[40] Metis and non-status Indians, including at least some of Brian Sinclair's family, would not have been counted in these figures. A 1959 provincial study estimated that about 3,500 people who identified as "Metis or Half-Breed" lived in the city.[41] Between 1961 and 2006, the proportion of Indigenous people residing in urban areas in Canada grew from 13 to 53 percent. Between 2001 and 2006, Winnipeg's Indigenous population increased 23 percent; by 2006 it numbered 68,385, the largest of any major Canadian city.[42]

This growth was about more than people moving from reserve to city. Mary Jane Norris and Stewart Clatworthy's careful studies of patterns of migration for Indigenous people in the last half of the twentieth century make clear that the narrative of

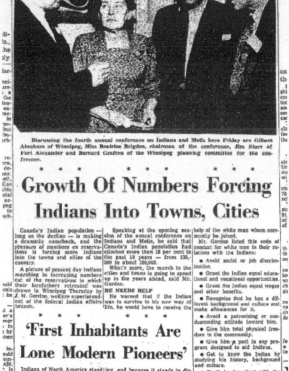

Discussing the fourth annual conference on Indians and Metis here Friday are Gilbert Abraham of Winnipeg, Miss Beatrice Brigden, chairman of the conference, Jim Starr of Fort Alexander and Bernard Grafton of the Winnipeg planning committee for the conference.

* * * * * * *

Growth Of Numbers Forcing Indians Into Towns, Cities

Canada's Indian population — long on the decline — is making a dramatic comeback, and the pressure of numbers on reservations is forcing more Indians into the towns and cities of the country.

A picture of present day Indians marching in increasing numbers out of the reservations to which their forefathers retreated was drawn in Winnipeg Thursday by J. H. Gordon, welfare experimentent of the federal Indian affairs branch.

Speaking at the opening session of the annual conference on Indians and Metis, he said that Canada's Indian population had climbed more than 18 per cent in the past 10 years — from 135,000 to about 200,000.

What's more, the march in the cities and towns is going to speed up in the years ahead, said Mr. Gordon.

HE NEEDS HELP

He warned that if the Indian was to survive in his new way of life, he would have to receive the help of the white man whom community be joined.

Mr. Gordon listed this code of conduct for white men in their relations with the Indians:

● Avoid social or job discrimination.

● Grant the Indian equal educational and vocational opportunities.

● Grant the Indian equal wages and other benefits.

● Recognize that he has a different background and culture and make allowances for it.

● Avoid a patronizing or condescending attitude toward him.

● Give him total physical freedom in the community.

● Give him a part in any program designed to aid Indians.

● Get to know the Indian by studying his history, background and culture.

● Don't be impatient with the

* * * * * * *

'First Inhabitants Are Lone Modern Pioneers'

Indians of North America stand alone as "twentieth century pioneering, and because it stands in direct contrast with former work-

Figure 8. A 1958 article of the *Winnipeg Free Press* "Growth of Numbers Forcing Indians into Towns, Cities" discusses population growth and urbanization of Indigenous people following the Second World War as it reports on the fourth annual conference of the Indian and Metis Committee of the Community Welfare Planning Council of Winnipeg.

reserve-to-city cannot fully explain the shape and pace of the growth of urban Indigenous populations. Focusing on twelve cities, including Winnipeg, they demonstrate that the impact of net in-migration (that is, Indigenous people moving *to* the city minus those leaving it) was the greatest between 1966 and 1971. Thereafter, the role of migration was reduced and, importantly, "variable in direction": Indigenous people moved to the city, but they also left it. Natural increase was a "significant contributor" to population growth in Winnipeg. Legislative changes and what Norris and Clatworthy call "ethnic mobility/drift," or changes in how people identify over time, also account for the sustained growth of Indigenous populations in Canadian cities, including Winnipeg.[43]

In one way or another, the segregated social order that had developed in the Canadian West was remade in the last third of the twentieth century, and Winnipeg was re-Indigenized, though on distinctly unequal and spacialized terms. Non-Indigenous journalists, scholars, and observers who wrote about what they called the "urban Indian problem" of the postwar era, as Leslie Hall has noted, tended to frame the very existence of urban Indigenous people as a problem unto itself, and the troubles they encountered as largely of their own making.[44] They also cast it in distinctly cultural terms. "The primary cause of the problems faced by the Indian and Metis is a cultural one," explained Jean Lagassé,

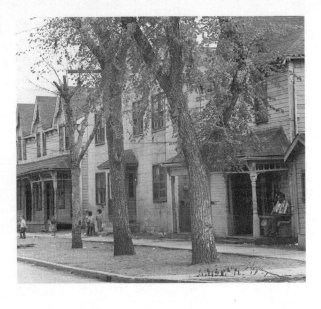

Figure 9. By the 1960s, sizeable parts of
Winnipeg's core had become home to Indigenous
people. Here, Joe Desjarlais sits on his porch on
Jarvis Street in 1963 while kids play on a July day.

an official in Manitoba's Department of Welfare: "Their culture was not designed for a western industrial world."[45]

The patterns of segregation that defined First Nations and settler histories in western Canada were remade *within* the city. More than 73 percent of Indigenous people studied in a 1970 doctoral dissertation lived within the "primary core area" of Winnipeg.[46] More than three decades later, there were ten census areas in Winnipeg where Indigenous people made up 30 percent or more of the total population, and one in which they accounted for more than half. The concentration of Indigenous people in poor neighbourhoods in Winnipeg's centre was still high, both in literal terms and compared with other Canadian cities.[47]

While academic studies have placed (and sometimes continue to place) primary weight on the material and economic circumstances that drive these patterns, they have also examined the way that social boundaries were produced and maintained through spatial practices of racism and segregation that kept Indigenous people out of certain areas, even if they had the money or the inclination to relocate. A 1959 study enumerated some of the de facto practices of segregation that Indigenous people in Winnipeg met with: for instance, landlords redirected potential tenants to less desirable apartments or neighbourhoods, and hotelkeepers either would not accept Indigenous guests or "would prefer not to."[48] More than a decade later, Don McCaskill's 1970 dissertation found that Indigenous people, when asked, reported that "discrimination" was the part of Winnipeg life they were "most distressed" about. Interviewees singled out being directly discriminated against by "landlords, taxi drivers, and sales clerks."[49]

Practices of segregation were sometimes overt. The Manitoba Liquor Act passed in 1928 specified that liquor permits were necessary for people to enter beer parlours, and such permits would not be issued to "any Indian or interdicted person."[50] Here, as elsewhere, restricted access to bars and restaurants was clearly a type of informal and formal segregation. Revisions to the Indian Act in 1951 meant that status Indians were no longer legally barred from access to alcohol, but, as Dale Barbour explains, it was up to the provinces to make changes to laws within their jurisdictions. In 1955 Manitoba published the *Report of the Manitoba Liquor Enquiry Commission*, which othered Indigenous people, imagined them as male, and regularly suggested that Indigenous people inherently lacked the capacity to manage liquor.[51]

In 1962, a journalist from the *Winnipeg Free Press* reported that "Winnipeg hasn't the segregated seating found in some rural Manitoba beer parlours, it lacks the separate entrances and seats of Indians to the right, whites to the left, found in the theatre at Pine Falls," but acknowledged that "in the city the segregation is imposed by basic economies in housing, jobs, and entertainment."[52] Yet speaking of patterns and practices of segregation, informal or formal, remained (and remains) a complicated social act in mainstream circles in Winnipeg. In 1987 Metis leader Audreen Hourie "touched a sensitive nerve" when she called attention to "informal segregation in Winnipeg schools," arguing that Indigenous children were "being gathered together and given a second-rate education."[53]

The history of Indigenous people in Winnipeg in the postwar era is much more than one of loss. It is also a history of remarkable community-building and resistance. One of its premier organizations was the Indian and Metis Friendship Centre (IMFC), which opened in 1959. As Hall notes, the Indigenous founders of the IMFC firmly rejected the contention that Indigenous culture was incompatible with urban life, and instead pointed to the barriers of systematic racism, underfunding, and colonization.[54] The late 1960s and 1970s witnessed the increased presence of and legal and practical access to a range of modes of Indigenous protest, and the growth of the Red Power movement.[55] The City of Winnipeg's Community and Race Relations Committee, established in 1981, initially prioritized the issues and concerns of racialized migrants, but its work with groups like the Winnipeg Council of Treaty Indians, as McCallum has noted elsewhere, points to the long history of ways that people have "acknowledged discrimination, documented and defined prejudice and imagined alternatives" for Indigenous people in the city.[56]

In 1972, a coalition of twenty-one Indigenous organizations joined together to form Neeginan, a community services centre that would provide accommodation for Indigenous organizations and agencies. Neeginan became a focal point for "social and cultural life of the Native community."[57] Research into Winnipeg's Indigenous institutional history in the 1970s and 1980s documents the variety of organizations and efforts to provide services and opportunities to Indigenous people that would, critically, be delivered by Indigenous people and reflect Indigenous priorities.[58]

The Indigenous music scene of the 1960s and 1970s, with bands like the Feathermen and C-Weed based in bars on the Main Street strip and featured at events at the IMFC, reflected both the segregated character of Winnipeg that penetrated even its arts scene and the rich Indigenous culture that developed in the teeth of struggle. "We didn't pursue white venues because we knew we'd have the door slammed in our faces," explained Anishinaabe blues musician Billy Joe Green. "We came from the streets and had experienced the apartheid that existed."[59] The Professional Native Indian Artists, colloquially known as the Indian Group of Seven, was established in Winnipeg in the early 1970s by seven painters, including Daphne Odjig and Jackson Beardy.[60] In literature, the work of a new generation of Indigenous authors, including novelist Beatrice Culleton Mosionier and poet Duncan Mercredi, described urban Indigenous experience in new and vivid terms.[61]

The population growth and the enduring patterns of inequality and exclusion fuelled what we might call a North End renaissance, a cultural explosion that started in the 1960s and continued well into the 1990s and 2000s. The 2016 census found that Winnipeg had more than 90,000 people identifying as First Nations, Metis, or Inuit, which translates to a little over 12 percent of the total population.[62] Older Indigenous organizations, like the food sovereignty project Neechi Foods, grew and consolidated. New organizations were formed, including Ka Ni Kanichihk, which was established in 2002. It would go on to play a critical role in the response to Brian Sinclair's death.

In the 1990s and 2000s Indigenous people had made a particular mark on the city and the province's electoral politics. Status Indians who lived on reserve and collected treaty annuities could not vote in provincial elections in Manitoba until 1952, and status Indians could not vote federally until 1960. In the years following the franchise, Manitoba elected some prominent Indigenous politicians, including Elijah Harper (1949–2013), Oscar Lathlin (1947–2008), and Eric Robinson (b. 1953). Indigenous candidates, whose election to provincial and federal offices had largely been confined to northern parts of the province, were now being elected in the city. Brian Bowman, who identifies as Metis, was elected Winnipeg's mayor in 2014, the first Indigenous mayor of a major Canadian city.[63] According to political scientist Kiera Ladner, Indigenous voter participation surged in the 2014 municipal election and in the 2015 federal election.[64] It was less robust in the provincial election of 2016, but the strong presence of Indigenous, urban MLAs—Kevin Chief and then Bernadette Smith for Point Douglas, Nahanni Fontaine for St. John's, and Wab Kinew for Fort Rouge— suggests a shift in the electoral politics of the city's most Indigenous precincts.

Mainstream journalists and analysts have struggled to explain a place that was, simultaneously, both so Indigenous and so clearly organized along lines of race and exclusion. Scholars have puzzled over whether Winnipeg conformed to American experiences of ghettoization, noting that in 2001 one in five people in Winnipeg's inner city identified themselves as Indigenous, while only one in twenty outside of it did.[65] A local journalist tried to explain the city to an international audience by describing it as a place facing a "great indigenous divide" in 2014. A year later, a national Canadian magazine, *Maclean's,* described Winnipeg as the place "where Canada's racism problem is at its worst."[66]

It is within this context that Brian Sinclair spent his last thirty-four hours in 2008. His was one of a cluster of tragic deaths of Indigenous people that garnered attention, outrage, and sorrow, and triggered discussions about what colonialism has meant and continues to mean in Canadian cities. In the summer of 2014, Tina Fontaine, a member of the Sagkeeng First Nation, where Brian Sinclair also had history and ties, was found dead in the Red River. Fontaine's death, which is one of many being examined by the National Inquiry into Murdered and Missing Indigenous Women and Girls, became a painful and enduring lesson on the connections between violence and a dysfunctional child welfare system where Indigenous children are radically overrepresented. Stories like those of Tina Fontaine and Brian Sinclair can only make sense when we think about the long and ongoing histories of colonialism that have made and remade this difficult, complex place.

The statistics on Indigenous health, welfare, and mortality are readily available and rarely disputed. All across Canada, Indigenous people are disproportionately poor and disproportionately likely to find themselves incarcerated or caught up in the child welfare system. Indigenous women are nearly three times more likely than non-Indigenous women to be victims of a violent crime; the homicide rate for Indigenous women is seven times higher than that of non-Indigenous women and, as research on Saskatchewan shows, up to 60 percent of missing women are Indigenous.[67] Indigenous people are much more likely than the Canadian population as a whole to suffer ill health, and on average Indigenous people do not live nearly as long as non-Indigenous Canadians. None of this is news to Indigenous people, nor to Canadians and their governments. Non-Indigenous Canada has cyclically discovered and rediscovered a problem that has become framed as a crisis of Indigenous Canada, prompting new and deeply familiar waves of attention and promises. As Pamela Palmater argues, "The fact that racism against Indigenous people generally, and Indigenous women and girls specifically, has been normalized does not mean that society is not aware of the problem. There is no level of government today—federal, provincial, territorial, municipal— that can deny that Canada has a serious racism problem, one that is killing Indigenous people."[68]

This recitation of terrible facts testifying to the continued immiseration, incarceration, and diminution of Indigenous people does not tell the whole story of Indigenous life, in Winnipeg or elsewhere, in all its layers, its tenacity, and its richness. These numbers can and often do sensationalize. The numbers also generalize, rendering invisible the Indigenous people who enjoy good health and live long lives, and who, as individuals, families, and communities, manage to navigate a world that is not of their own making. But for all of this, these measures tell us something important about modern Canadian colonialism, now more than a century-and-a-half old, how it works, and what it has taken and continues to take from Indigenous people. Jaskiran Dhillon explains that "colonial power depends on the systematic redefinition and transformation of the terrain upon which the life of the colonized is lived," whether it is the forced removal to residential schools, the "ostensibly rehabilitative incarceration," or the regulation of identity and kinship through the Indian Act.[69] The institution of the hospital, including the one where Brian Sinclair spent his last thirty-four hours, is another manifestation of this colonial power, and of the lethal racism and the structures of indifference that it both produces and depends on.

THE HOSPITAL

2

THE STRUCTURES OF INDIFFERENCE WE examine in this book are registered in a range of places in Canada's past and present. This chapter focuses on hospitals, and in particular Winnipeg's Health Sciences Centre, where Brian Sinclair spent his last hours in 2008. However, hospitals are part of a range of institutional systems in Canada shaped by settler colonialism, Indigenous dispossession and marginalization, Canadian nation-state building in the nineteenth century, and the maintenance of white settler prosperity and priority through the twentieth and twenty-first. For more than a century, from the 1880s when the federal government began to fund Indian residential schools (IRS), to the 1990s when the last IRS closed, residential schools for Indigenous children were a vivid and enduring example of Canada's colonial and often carceral relations with Indigenous people.[1] Our present-day child welfare systems, especially in the western provinces, have raised similar problems. In 2017, it was reported that up to 90 percent of children "in care" in Manitoba were Indigenous, and even the federal minister of Indigenous Services noted that these circumstances were "very much reminiscent of the residential school system."[2] Similar connections can be and are routinely made about the criminal justice systems. In Manitoba, the Aboriginal Justice Inquiry (AJI) in 1991 found that Indigenous people accounted for more than half of the prisoners in Manitoba's correctional institutions.[3] Some thirty years later, the figures are more rather than less startling. As many as nine in ten women at Manitoba's Women's Correctional Centre in Headingley are Indigenous, and Indigenous men make up 65 percent of the inmate population in the federal Stony Mountain Institution. Many are there because of failing to comply with a curfew or bail conditions or because they were charged with a low-level drug offence and are serving mandatory-minimum sentences.[4]

Hospitals are not jails, foster homes, or residential schools. Yet hospitals have a particular place within the network of institutions and institutional practices that continue to regulate, and not infrequently imperil, Indigenous lives in settler colonial Canada. The particular history of Winnipeg's HSC, where Brian Sinclair spent his last thirty-four hours, is the subject of this chapter. It speaks to the connections between health care and settler colonialism, and to the complicated ways that hospitals are experienced by those who live in Manitoba and Winnipeg.

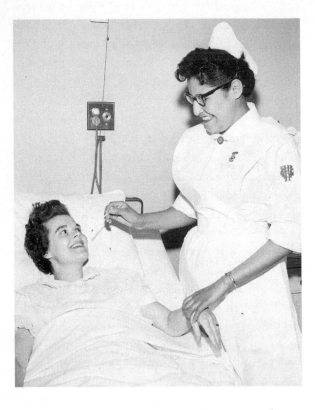

Figure 10. Nurse Ann Thomas Callahan at
work at the Winnipeg General Hospital in
1960.

The HSC is located in what is both an unmistakably Indigenous and enduringly colonial place. The building that houses the ER waiting room where Brian Sinclair died is called the Ann Thomas Building (see Figure 11). Ann Thomas Callahan was one of the first Indigenous people to graduate from the nursing program at the Winnipeg General Hospital (WGH), now the HSC.[5] The building, opened in 2007, was the largest health care capital project in Manitoba history, and it honours Thomas's "lifelong dedication to healing, wellness and learning."[6] Thomas was raised in a rich and loving family at Peepeekisis Cree Nation, Saskatchewan before spending fourteen years in residential schools, including File Hills Indian Residential School and Birtle Residential School, some 200 kilometres away in southern Manitoba. She then moved another 300 kilometres east to Winnipeg to study and work as a nurse in the 1950s. Helping to create the first Indigenous professional organization, the Registered Nurses of Canadian Indian Ancestry (now Indigenous Nurses Association of Canada) in the 1970s, she was also involved in educating health professionals at Winnipeg's Red River College from 1983 to her retirement in 1996. According to the Winnipeg Regional Health Authority, "In her commitment to healthcare, community and continuous learning, Ann Thomas Callahan embodies the spirit that defines Health Sciences Centre Winnipeg."[7] Callahan is a well-known elder in Winnipeg, and her own life history reflects profoundly important and ongoing equity issues in Indigenous education, labour, and health, as well as a desire to acknowledge Indigenous women's contribution to health care and the history of Winnipeg and of Canada. Her name on the building is a reminder of the visibility—and invisibility—of Indigenous people within Canadian health care systems.

Moving out from the Ann Thomas building, many other places in and around the HSC campus also reflect the hospital's rootedness in local Indigenous and colonial history. Several of the buildings are named after white settler doctors, nurses, and donors. The Isabel M. Stewart building was named for one of the leading North American nurse educators of her time. She was one of many late nineteenth- and early twentieth-century health care professionals (including her brother, D.A. Stewart, a celebrated Manitoba physician noted for his treatment of tuberculosis) who came from Protestant English or Scottish families and moved to Manitoba from Ontario for a variety of reasons, including Christian missionary work, the lure of land, and opportunities to work in the medical field. The Chown Building is named after Henry Havelock Chown, a physician, surgeon, professor, and dean of the Manitoba Medical College. Chown also became chief medical officer of the Great West Life Assurance Company; his son Bruce researched the mechanism of Rh disease. The

Brodie Centre is named after Earle and Marion Brodie, a physician and nurse couple who partnered with Sol Price in founding retail giants FedMart and the Price Club, the original cash-and-carry membership warehouse, and who made a substantial gift to the University of Manitoba. The Thorlakson Building was named after a surgeon and medical educator of Icelandic and Norwegian descent, Paul H.T. Thorlakson, who practised briefly at Shoal Lake, Manitoba, and helped found the Winnipeg Clinic. The Kleysen Institute is named after Dutch-Canadian businessman and philanthropist Hubert Kleysen, of the successful transportation, distribution, and industrial products company. The Cadham Lab was named after Dr. Fred T. Cadham, who, along with Dr. Gordon Bell, was one of the first prominent bacteriologists and hygienists in the province. From London, Ontario, Cadham's father in 1870 had answered Canada's call to arms to subdue Metis resistance at Red River. He volunteered in the Red River Expedition under General Wolseley, and he decided to stay after his discharge and became an architect.[8] The John Buhler Research Centre is named after the farm machinery entrepreneur and health and education philanthropist with roots in the Russian Mennonite community based in Morden, Manitoba. Settling in 1874 in the "West Reserve," this group was attracted by promises of "free land" in a white settlement scheme that followed on the tail

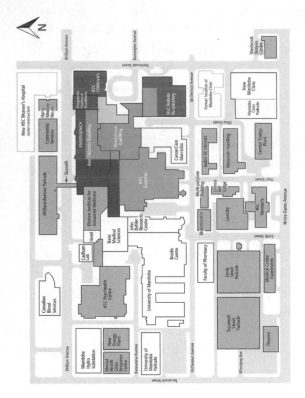

Figure 11. Winnipeg's Health Sciences Centre in 2018.

of the signing of Treaty 1; it involved territory that had been promised to Metis communities after the resistance (see Figure 6). This and other settlement schemes hastened the removal of First Nations and Metis people from desirable agricultural land.[9]

The street names around the Health Sciences Centre also speak to the city's history and the context in which the hospital itself was built. Of these streets, McDermot, Bannatyne, and Tecumseh[10] dominated the original site and continue to be main thoroughfares for those visiting and working at the HSC. McDermot and Bannatyne streets trace the land holdings of elite HBC fur traders and Red River families who will be examined more closely later in this chapter. Tecumseh Street, the western boundary of the HSC, references a different place and time and was likely named in commemoration of the War of 1812, but also evokes a history of British loyalty, colonialism, the Canadian nation, and Indigenous death and decline (see Figure 11). Local historian Harry Shave exclaimed, "It is fitting that in the name of a Winnipeg street, bordering an institution of help and comfort in suffering humanity, the memory of Tecumseh should be perpetuated."[11] Indeed, this is one of many examples by which Tecumseh's name was "co-opted" to reinforce righteous narratives of white settler colonialism and Canadian nation-building.[12]

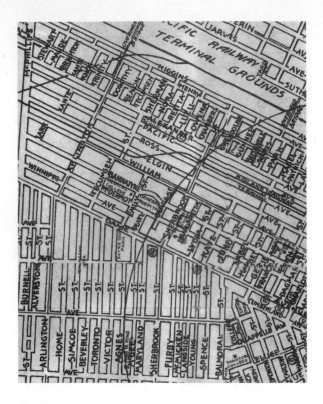

Figure 12. This 1919 map shows the streets
in and around the Winnipeg General Hospital
(now HSC).

Other street names in the area, including William, Sherbrook, Notre Dame, Pearl, Emily, and Olivia,[13] like many of the streets in the city as a whole, are landmarks of nation- and city-builders and defenders—retired fur-trade company agents and officers, military men, land owners and speculators, businessmen, and their wives and daughters. Some streets were named after Hudson's Bay Company (HBC), Metis, and First Nations families who built a significant network for commerce, land ownership, and governance in the nineteenth century.[14]

To acknowledge the long history of the HSC is to understand that its development relied profoundly on the transfer of Indigenous lands, funds, and labour and that this transfer did not cease with the HBC claim to Rupertsland, nor was it symbolic or always involuntary. The HSC's institutional and spatial history is linked directly to two prominent Winnipeg families, the McDermots and the Bannatynes, each tied to Indigenous lineages through women. Andrew McDermot and his wife Sarah (McNab) granted land title for the present-day HSC campus,[15] and Andrew Bannatyne, the McDermots' son-in-law, also made a land donation. Both McDermot and Bannatyne were second-generation HBC men who had likely obtained their land upon retiring from the company and, by extension, through the HBC's particular colonial claim to title of Rupertsland. Andrew McDermot was born in Ireland and joined the

HBC in his youth, arriving in York Factory in 1812. He married Sarah Mary McNab, a Metis woman from Berens River, *à la façon du pays*, or by Indigenous rite, a few years later at Norway House, and together they had fifteen surviving children. When McDermot retired with his family to Red River, he became a merchant and later joined the local governing Council of Assiniboia in 1839.[16]

Andrew Bannatyne was a fur trader and merchant from Orkney who entered HBC service in 1846, stationed in Norway House. A few years later, he married the McDermots' daughter Annie and went into business in Red River, building a large merchant firm. Bannatyne was also a member of the Council of Assiniboia, supported Riel and A.D. Lepine during the 1869–70 Resistance, and was a member of the short-lived North-West Council (1870–76). He also served as postmaster and was a Freemason, member of the Manitoba Club, and a founding member of the Manitoba Historical Society. Andrew and Annie (McDermot) Bannatyne had ten children.

Annie Bannatyne was a community leader and philanthropist in Red River, known for her hospitality and skill in hosting charitable functions. She and the local Ladies Association are credited with raising substantial funds for the initial hospital building and furnishings. The value of such work should not be underestimated. In 1873, Annie Bannatyne

The Title Deed.

"To have and to hold unto the said parties of the third part" (the Winnipeg general hospital) "and their assigns to and for their sole and only use forever subject to the provisions hereinafter contained. Provided always, and these presents are upon this express condition, that the said parties of the third part shall within two years after the date hereof enact and establish a hospital on the said lands and premises and shall use and occupy the said lands and premises for the purpose immediately connected with such hospital exclusively. And provided, further, should the said parties of the third part at any time hereafter consider it desirable and advantageous to sell or otherwise dispose of the said land and premises and to erect a hospital building elsewhere then the whole proceeds arising from such sale or disposition shall be applied towards the erection and establishment of such new hospital and the support and maintenance thereof. But provided always that the purchaser or purchasers thereof shall in no wise be held liable or responsible for the due application of the purchase money aforesaid. The said party of the first part hereby releases to the said parties of the third part all his claims upon this said lands and premises subject to the provisions above contained."

Figure 13. In 1910, Andrew and Sarah McDermot's donation of lands for the Winnipeg General Hospital was commemorated in the city's daily newspaper.

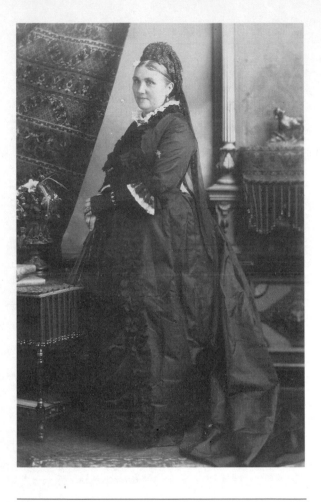

Figure 14. Red River daughter and Winnipeg philanthropist and community organizer Annie McDermot Bannatyne (c. 1830–1908). This photo was taken in Montreal in 1882.

organized two bazaars that raised $1,700 and $950, respectively, for the new hospital.[17] Another bazaar in September 1874 also raised funds for the hospital.[18] Historian Norma Hall points out that in 1875, the same year that Annie applied for scrip for herself and her children, Mrs. Bannatyne and Mrs. Hector McKenzie handed over $1,345.80 to help fund the hospital by hosting a series of summer bazaars and concerts.[19] The Ladies Association eventually became the Women's Hospital Aid Association, continuing to organize fundraising bazaars and balls to supply the hospital with bedding, clothing, and other necessities. The Winnipeg General Hospital itself, Hall argues, is an "enduring legacy, extended by Anne [Annie] to people well beyond the limits of her circle of friends and family" (see Figures 13 and 14).[20]

Elite and middle-class women in late-nineteenth-century Winnipeg often played a central role in raising funds and organizing efforts to build institutions such as hospitals and schools. While women were largely excluded from formal participation in political life, care for the sick and education of youth were seen as predominantly their domain well into the twentieth century. This work was carried out by paid nursing and teaching staff as well as through voluntary labour of church and other women's groups, many of whom sought to influence public health laws and policies and to support the founding and functioning of hospitals and schools.

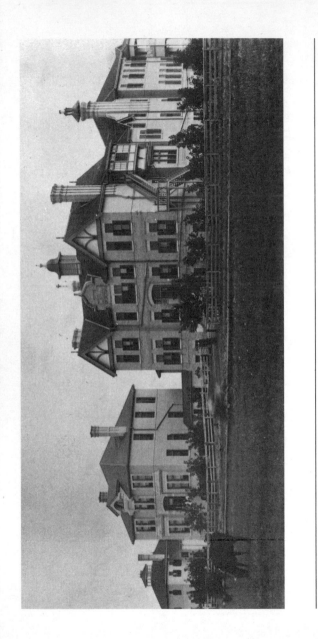

Figure 15. The visually impressive Winnipeg General Hospital, around 1893.

This work was very much part of the everyday life and social network in Red River/Winnipeg in the 1870s. For example, the *Manitoba Free Press* reported on one of the bazaars, held in August 1873, as "A Magnificent Affair—Remembering the Sick." The two-day bazaar, in aid of the erection of the WGH, was held in the Red River court room, which had been "thoroughly cleared of all the administration of justice furniture . . . [and replaced by] rainbow hued drapery spangles, flags and evergreens. The room was most tastefully decorated, a score of Union Jacks being suspended from the wall, interspersed with evergreens, flowers and other ornaments" [and] the words "remember the sick" were beautifully twined in evergreens. . . . The tables were well supplied with a great variety of all the odds and ends, and useful and ornamental articles which are generally to be found in similar places and the fair saleswomen acquitted themselves in a manner which would put to shame the efforts of some of our first class male professional counter-jumping friends. Refreshments, too, could be had, and the conventional bazaar concomitants of a post office, grab bag, lotteries, auctions and other mild and tolerated swindles were there in abundance and created in the usual quantity of merriment." There was a ball on the first evening, and the newspaper reported the hall to be "crowded with richly dressed ladies and amiable looking gentlemen," entertained by "the sweet strains of the military band."

At the end of the second day, the bazaar was brought to a close with ceremonies, and gratitude was extended to the ladies who, "through a great deal of labour and expense so well succeeded in doing so much for a most praiseworthy object at the same time that they afforded opportunity and enjoyment."[21]

Annie McDermot, the women she worked with, and the larger community at Red River wanted a hospital for a variety of reasons. The hospital was proposed and initiated to address medical needs brought about by military conflict, poor sanitation, flooding, the pollution of rivers, and the spread of tuberculosis, venereal disease, smallpox, diphtheria, and scarlet fever. A substantial number of the WGH's early patients were treated for typhoid, also known as "Red River Fever," a common disease at the time, often associated with drinking contaminated water directly from the Red River. Typhoid would continue to be a major health concern until the city of Winnipeg, with the help of the Indian Affairs department, confiscated land at Shoal Lake 40 First Nation in the early twentieth century in order to build an aqueduct that would carry clean water to the city of Winnipeg.[22] The hospital's early years are also closely connected to the uprising of Metis and allied First Nations and settlers in the Northwest Resistance of 1885, as surgeons at the WGH "rallied to the cause," helping to organize teams of surgeons and medical students to assist at hospitals in Saskatoon,

Battleford, and Moose Jaw. In addition, injured soldiers were transferred back to special wards at the WGH.[23] The hospital was built to treat those living at Red River; increasingly however, as the population at Red River and Winnipeg shifted, the hospital came to serve a population of city dwellers that was less and less Indigenous.[24]

While modern medicine is often depicted as being at odds with Indigenous medicine, Indigenous and non-Indigenous people shared a desire for ready access to modern health care facilities. Indigenous people adapted and combined different approaches to medicine even as Christian missionaries and other authorities sought to prohibit all but normative medical practices. This included not only the ongoing practice of plant medicine, midwifery, ceremony, and dance but also, where possible, efforts to critically shape and influence modern health care.[25] And yet access to health care was not equally available to all, and in fact the history of modern medicine in Manitoba was deeply invested in racial segregation—and vice versa. As historian Ryan Eyford shows, the management of the public health crisis of smallpox in 1876–77 by quarantine dovetailed with efforts to remove Cree, Anishinaabeg, and Metis people from around the southern basin of Lake Winnipeg and to isolate them on Indian reserves and land reserved for "half-breeds."[26] The management of another racialized epidemic close on its tail, this time of tuberculosis, was also acutely influential, as political jurisdictions fought over who was responsible for First Nations care and if and how that care would be justified.

From the late nineteenth century to the first half of the twentieth century, tuberculosis became a major public health concern in Canada and elsewhere. While tuberculosis was present throughout society in western Canada at all levels and in all places, many more Indigenous than non-Indigenous people had active, serious, and deadly cases of the disease. This led to the widespread assumption that people of Indigenous ancestry were racially susceptible to the disease. In fact, major risk factors for tuberculosis include dislocation, poverty, malnutrition, overcrowding, and inadequate housing, conditions experienced at this time by large segments of the First Nations and Metis populations in Manitoba. These circumstances are direct outcomes of colonization, and of repressive economic, political, cultural, and social policies, military invasions, dispossession and white settlement, and the loss of natural resources. Nonetheless, at the time medical experts in the province and elsewhere concluded that Indigenous people were biologically and racially susceptible to disease and posed a terrible danger (or "menace," in D.A. Stewart's view)[27] to white citizens who might come into contact with them. A system of segregated health care in Canada consolidated amid the perceived threat of "Indian tuberculosis."

At the time, TB treatment involved isolating contagious patients at sanatoria, special hospitals where patients had access to fresh air, good nutrition, rest, and surgery if necessary. Ninette, the first sanatorium in Manitoba, opened in 1910. This sanatorium, however, did not serve Indigenous patients until the mid-twentieth century, after the disease had come under control among the white population. That health care institutions in Canada worked to "protect" white settlers from Indigenous people conflicts with mainstream ideas about the history of Canada's health care system. As historian Maureen Lux argues, this segregated care "made it seemingly natural that the sanatorium and the modernizing hospital would be reserved for white patients."[28]

Indigenous people with tuberculosis were isolated on reserves and treated within an ad hoc and half-hearted medical service provided by school and field nurses and fee-for-service physicians hired by the Department of Indian Affairs (DIA). Or the sick were simply ignored and left to get sicker and die, as one official pointed out in 1907. In an important moment of resistance in Indigenous health services history, then chief medical officer of the DIA, Dr. Peter Bryce, published a report on the extent of tuberculosis in Indian residential schools and roundly criticized the institutions and the DIA for contributing to the spread of the disease among Indigenous people. He reported, "of a total of 1,537 pupils reported upon nearly 25 percent are dead, of one school with an absolutely accurate statement, 69 percent of ex-pupils are dead, and that everywhere the almost invariable cause of death given is tuberculosis."[29] Bryce appealed to the government to increase spending to help address the high death and disease rates of children in the schools. However, his recommendations contradicted the policy to reduce funding to Indian health outlined by Duncan Campbell Scott, Deputy Superintendent of the DIA, and Scott blocked Bryce's critical research on the schools and its dissemination. The DIA did not have a chief medical officer again until 1927, when E.L. Stone became head of the new, separate medical branch within Indian Affairs. At that time, the DIA confidently reported that it was responsible for "all matters appertaining to health of Indians."[30]

Only after sustained pressure did the federal government commit funds to address tuberculosis among Indigenous people.[31] Still, the federal government has consistently held that "neither law nor treaty" compels it to provide health services to First Nations, indicating rather that this function was a "moral obligation." However, health care was part of discussions of the numbered treaties in western Canada. The only treaty to specifically refer to medical care is Treaty 6 (in medicine chest and pestilence clauses); however, promises relating to health were made during the negotiations of other treaties. In addition, because treaties were negotiated at a time in which Indigenous health had been put in extreme peril—in circumstances amounting to genocide—and because vaccinations and other types of medical care were distributed at annual meetings where treaty annuities were paid, health care was indelibly linked to the treaty relationship.[32] In many places, health services were seen as rightfully belonging to communities, and as representing the sacred and legal relationship between the Crown and sovereign Indigenous nations that entails continued obligations for both parties. What health care was offered, however, was designed on a self-serving model characterized by parsimony and moral sanctity: limited, often ineffectual, medical and nursing services, funded and delivered unequally and separately, ensured that Canadian medicine would support the health of Canadian settlers first and foremost.

The creation and development of Indian Health Services occurred within a structure of colonial power that included the Indian Act, DIA management philosophy, tools of coercion (including withholding of treaty annuities and other benefits), and federal law enforcement that ensured that First Nations people could be (and were) compelled to obey the bizarre and ever-changing regulations of Indian Health Services. For example, in addition to provincial health laws, First Nations people were subject to special health regulations, adapted into the Indian

Act. Amendments to the Act in 1953, for example criminalized the refusal to see a doctor, go to hospital, or leave a hospital before discharge. The Royal Canadian Mounted Police could and did arrest First Nations patients and returned them to hospitals or sent them to prison.[33]

Outside of DIA services, Indigenous people were by and large refused at municipal and provincial hospitals, or they were treated in segregated and basement wards and wings that were substandard to the rest of the hospital. In part, this was because the DIA refused to pay for hospital care at the same rate as Canadians paid. Such a view that health care for Indigenous people should be cheaper, and by extension lesser, than that offered to Canadians remained a core principle of Indian Health Services, even as it moved into an era of developing hospitals and health care centres in the 1940s and 1950s. These "Indian Hospitals" operated by the federal government are testament to a history of racial segregation, systemic discrimination in health care, inferior treatment, and health inequity.

The history of hospitals located in the communities that Brian Sinclair and his family were connected to helps to illuminate this disparity and racial segregation in health care. Until the late 1930s, Indigenous people had very little access to health service, and this was especially problematic because of the virulent spread of tuberculosis. In 1937, a "preventorium" was constructed as part of the Fort Alexander IRS; it was an effort to isolate students who had contagious cases of tuberculosis while keeping them at the school, but the experiment failed.[34] Between 1939 and 1956, the Department of Indian Affairs contracted with the Sanatorium Board of Manitoba to convert Dynevor Indian Hospital, a nineteenth-century Anglican mission hospital north of Selkirk, Manitoba, into a very basic fifty-bed tuberculosis sanatorium for the segregated treatment of First Nations and some Metis people from Manitoba, northwestern Ontario, and Saskatchewan (and later Inuit from the central Arctic). In addition, during the 1930s, Indian Affairs contracted a physician at the hospital in the adjacent town of Pine Falls to serve the Fort Alexander reserve. "Townspeople objected to their presence,"[35] however, and so in 1938 the government built an annex to house the Fort Alexander Indian Hospital, which operated alongside the Pine Falls Hospital for nearly thirty years.[36]

The town of Pine Falls was not simply "adjacent" to Sagkeeng First Nation, explains Bella Malo, née Guimond, the Aboriginal liaison interpreter at the present-day Pine Falls Health Complex.[37] Rather, the town was, and is, considered by many to be part of the reserve, and this had implications for the way that health care was delivered. In a complicated and underhanded process described more thoroughly in Chapter 3, a section of the reserve was "surrendered" to a private interest, the Manitoba Pulp and Paper Company, in the 1920s and named Pine Falls. Pine Falls had its own hospital, owned and operated by the paper company until 1965. Completed in 1928 and renovated in 1952, the Pine Falls company hospital had a capacity of thirty beds and cribs. When the provincial Hospital Survey Board visited the hospital in 1960, Pine Falls Hospital had two full-time physicians and served about 3,600 people from the town of Pine Falls, the Rural Municipality of Powerview, and nearby communities—"exclusive of treaty Indians." At no point between 1955 and 1959 did Pine Falls Hospital ever record more than 43 percent occupancy.[38]

The Fort Alexander Indian Hospital, in contrast, had one doctor and a capacity of thirteen beds and three bassinets to serve the "Indian population east of Lake Winnipeg," including the Clandeboye Indian Agency, Fort Alexander, Little Black River, Hollow Water, Bloodvein, Berens River, and Little Grand Rapids—a total of approximately 2,600 people. When it was surveyed in 1960, it had set up twenty beds and five bassinets, even though this was beyond its physical and staff capacity. The Hospital Survey Board noted that the occupancy at Fort Alexander Indian Hospital ranged between 93 and 128 percent, a peak occupancy higher than any hospital of its size in the province.[39] This highlights the extent to which segregation and inequality was enforced in health care: underserviced First Nations

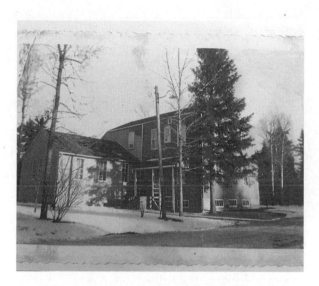

Figure 16. The Fort Alexander Indian Hospital in Pine Falls, Manitoba, opened in 1938, with an addition constructed in 1942. The hospital served Sagkeeng and surrounding First Nations.

people were literally turned away from open beds next door at Pine Falls. Moreover, not long after the Pine Falls Hospital was renovated, the survey board found Fort Alexander Indian Hospital to be unsafe and obsolete. While this example is unusual in that it involves a company-owned hospital, it was not unusual for Indian and non-Indian hospitals to be located close by, for there to be large gaps in service and standards, and for First Nations hospitals to be overcrowded while "mainstream" hospitals with more than enough resources turned First Nations patients away. The two hospitals amalgamated in 1965, were renovated in the 1980s, and now form part of the larger Pine Falls Health Complex site, which includes the Giigewigamig Traditional Healing Centre (opened in May 2017).

After the Second World War, a separate and growing system of health care for non-Indigenous people in Canada also gained momentum, but with much more funding and support. This system was accessible to status Indians only as an exception to the rule, with special permission from Indian agents required before health services could be accessed. There were many false and generalized justifications for this segregation—the most common was that First Nations people did not pay into the municipal or provincial tax base that funded community hospital construction and maintenance, though this argument self-servingly failed to note that public

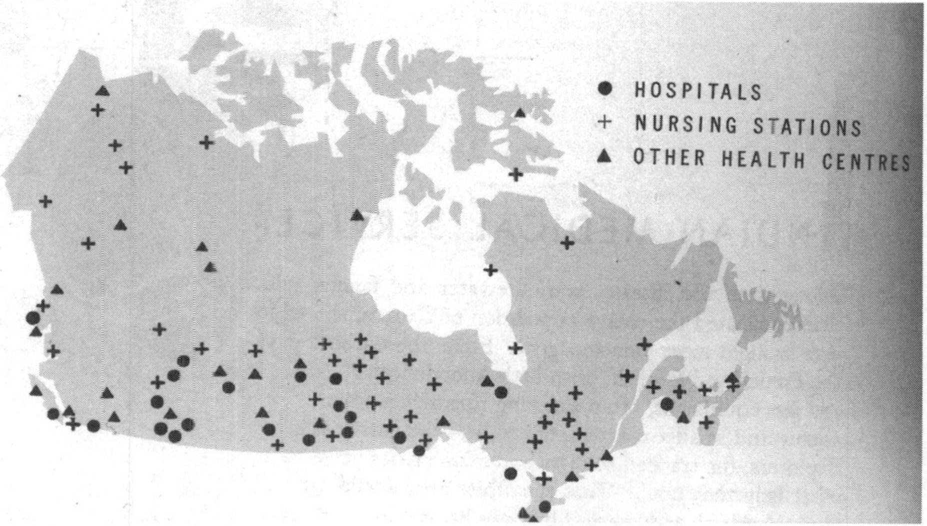

Figure 17. Map of Indian Health Services, 1961. Indian Health Services were planned and delivered by the federal government through a geographical division of the country into regions and zones with headquarters, superintendents, and medical officers.

HOSPITALS
NURSING STATIONS
OTHER HEALTH CENTRES

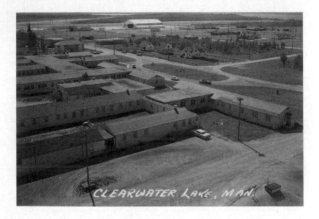

CLEARWATER LAKE, MAN.

Figure 18. Indian Health Services was paramilitary
in structure and closely connected to the actual military
in many places, such as the Clearwater Lake Indian
Hospital pictured here, which was a recycled U.S. air
force base erected during the Second World War near
The Pas, Manitoba.

hospitals like the HSC were in part funded by Indigenous money, situated on Indigenous land, and staffed with Indigenous labour, and that Indigenous people living off reserve paid many of the same taxes as non-Indigenous ones. In any event, many mainstream Canadians simply did not want to share a hospital with First Nations people, and this sentiment was protected and perpetuated by hospital administrations.

Despite these irregularities and inequities, we commonly speak of having a "universal health care system" in Canada, and in many ways our national identity is based on a collective pride in having free access to health care. However, the process by which medicare was implemented in Canada involved no consultation with Indigenous people, and yet had tremendous consequences for them. For example, prior to the introduction of medicare in 1968, the federal government gutted the Indian Health Services (IHS) budget under the auspices of "equality" and social and legal "integration" of First Nations within provincial health services. Under the new plan First Nations individuals could receive support for services only if they were proven to be indigent, had been refused band funds, and could not obtain provincial services. In addition, the federal government put a limit on IHS coverage to prevent "overutilization," and so diagnostic, outpatient, and preventive care were prioritized. Many First Nations saw this as an attempt to extinguish treaty rights to health care and forfeit federal responsibilities to Indigenous peoples. And indeed, the White Paper, a policy paper developed by the government of Pierre Elliott Trudeau that proposed to terminate all Indigenous rights and treaties in the name of "integration" and "equality," was tabled in medicare's wake, in 1969; it was roundly rejected by First Nations in short order. First Nations had additional concerns that in the context of provincial services, they would once again face discrimination, restricted access, and relegation to basement or segregated wards and "annexes." At the same time, many provincially funded community institutions saw Indigenous patients as a "burden best cared for by the federal government" in that they were non-tax-paying citizens and thus undeserving of provincial services. To access health care provision, Lux finds in her book on the history of Indian hospitals, members of First Nations were required to "exhaust all their resources before they would be helped, the very situation that Medicare presumably sought to remedy for other Canadians."[40] Discourses about rights such as universal health care that are meant to unite or create a supposed pan-Canadian experience or identity in actuality have failed to challenge colonial relations with Indigenous people and are, as historians Heidi Bohaker and Franca Iacovetta argue, "at odds with the historical reality of Canada."[41] As many First Nations feared, universal health care did not result in an improved experience for them; rather, prejudice and communication barriers in hospitals continued.

In line with contemporary liberal politics of multiculturalism in Canada more generally that encouraged respect for all and a welcoming of diversity, from the 1970s to the early 2000s, Winnipeg's HSC took some new approaches to service provision. For example, the traditional Christian chaplaincy program at the HSC extended more inclusive spiritual services, and health care providers—nurses, in particular—were trained to be "sensitive" to cultural differences between themselves and their patients, and to be "aware" of differences that could ultimately impact decisions about health care itself. Responding to ongoing problems in communication in particular with children of Indigenous families from the north, HSC created a Native Services Department in 1971, one of the first programs of its kind in Canada. According to Anishinaabe elder Margaret Lavallee, in the late 1970s the major functions of the department were written translation and oral interpretation services, including explaining consent forms and interpreting between doctors and patients. Lavallee, later the department's director, recalls that advocacy, facilitating dialogue, and translation were the main focus of their work: "Our goal was to build bridges between the two cultures and then on top of that to translate all of the medical terminology." In addition, the Native Services Department also helped to find clothing, accommodation, and food for visiting family members, and resources for patients and families after discharge.[42]

In November 1980, an incident at St. Boniface Hospital in Winnipeg brought national media attention to the treatment of Indigenous people in hospitals, and resulted in a number of recommendations to improve services. During a lung biopsy on a fifty-two-year-old woman from Shamattawa, in northern Manitoba, a surgeon tied glass beads into the ends of a suture. He later claimed he had joked about doing this with the patient, but that was not the case; in fact, she felt insulted and humiliated. The family involved the Assembly of Manitoba Chiefs (then called the Four Nations Confederacy), which wrote a brief with several important recommendations, including cultural awareness training, a twenty-four-hour program of interpreter and advocacy services for patients, and a formal administrative system that empowered staff to speak out when they saw patients mistreated and to seek investigations into patient complaints. In the inquiry into the complaint, Justice Emmett Hall supported these recommendations and acknowledged the breach of informed consent. In the end, however, Hall exonerated the surgeon of any racist and prejudiced intent, recommended that he not lose hospital privileges, and called the event "an error in judgment made with the best of intentions."[43] Hall did, however, stress that implementing recommendations meant to improve Indigenous patient experience required a serious commitment on the part of all medical staff, hospital personnel, and management.

In the early 1990s, the HSC was still struggling with this goal; it established an Aboriginal Services Review Committee to analyze if and how the HSC could better meet the needs of Indigenous people in Manitoba. In 1992 the committee released its report with several recommendations, including: increasing Indigenous representation on the HSC board of directors; increasing the autonomy and capacity of the Native Services Department; committing resources to ensure the availability of traditional healers for Indigenous patients; promoting employment equity and correcting the significant under-representation of Indigenous employees at the HSC;[44] establishing orientation and education programs to increase cultural awareness among employees of the HSC; improving community outreach activities and building relationships with Indigenous leaders in Manitoba; and increasing the number of Indigenous students in health professional educational programs.

It is significant that education is very much a part of these recommendations. The HSC has been, almost since its beginning, the central site for the training of physicians and nurses and for the production of knowledge about health and health care in Manitoba, as well as its largest hospital. Thus, the University of Manitoba Health Sciences complex has played a critical role in the development and delivery of modern racially segregated health care in the province. Dr. Percy E. Moore, who served as director of the Indian Health Services from 1946 to 1965 and heavily influenced Canadian postwar Indian health policy, graduated from the University of Manitoba's faculty of medicine. So, too, did countless others who worked in the Indian health system and who researched Indigenous health. These and other physicians would have been taught very little about Indigenous people; if they read medical and nursing journals, they would have learned that First Nations people were isolated, primitive, dependent, dirty, highly susceptible to disease, careless, childlike, and less evolved than whites.[45]

Such ideologies informed health research, policy decision-making, and treatment. As blatant notions of white supremacy fell out of favour in the postwar era, research based on "race" shifted to research based on "population," but retained many of the earlier methods and assumptions, including an emphasis on how biology, inherited traits, and now molecular genetics can explain inequities in health. Such a focus results in biased thinking in regard to diagnosis and treatment of "at risk" populations, while leaving underlying, and arguably far more significant and life-threatening, conditions unaddressed, and thus fails to acknowledge the legacy of colonialism and the complexity of individuals as human beings. Cree

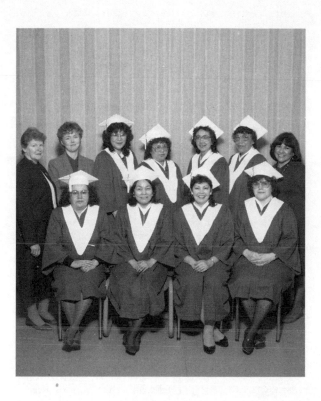

Figure 19.   Graduates of a Medical Interpreters course at the HSC Native Services Department in November 1986. As language specialists remind us, translation is not a straightforward process and involves subjective cultural and interpretive skills. Margaret Lavallee is standing at the far right.

scholar Jessica Kolopenuk asserts that indeed nine-teenth-century racial categories and logics continue to inform twenty-first-century biomedical research and that this research consistently fails to benefit the health of Indigenous people. Research remains focused on a search for a biological explanation of high TB morbidity rates among Indigenous people, leaving quite apart the colonial roots of health science, medicine, and research in Canada. She argues, "This consideration would necessitate inquiry into how constructing indigenous peoples as essentially fragile or inferior leads to narrow health care policies and bio-medical practices that target the supposedly pathological indigenous body, rather than the pathological colonial conditions which shape the political, socio-economic, ecological, and biological forces through which healthy and unhealthy bodies are produced."[46]

While "race" remains central to research on Indigenous health, "culture"—and specifically learning about presumably essential "Indigenous" culture, history, spirituality, "tradition" and "way of life"—has become a small part of revised curricula. However, Indigenous critical race scholars such as Linda Diffey argue that we would be much better served by anti-racist pedagogies that foreground an understanding of inequality as rooted in colonial power struggles, rather than in culture or ethnicity.[47]

The racialized logics found in Indigenous health research do not fit with the real and extraordinary ways in which Indigenous people have engaged—in many instances with little or no support and sometimes at their own peril—in efforts great and small to maintain and improve the health of their own people. The work of Indigenous communities is evident in hospitals and health centres, medical and nursing schools, research facilities, and professional and political organizations. Indigenous people have worked as cooks, cleaners, orderlies, and aides in hospitals and health centres across Canada, providing key support for the institutions and an important site of interaction with Indigenous patients. The health system has also relied heavily on the labour of translators and interpreters, who facilitate communication between patients, health care providers, and family members. Indigenous nurses and, although fewer in numbers, physicians, from at least the late nineteenth century on, have confronted barriers of language and educational backgrounds compromised by racism in Indian and mainstream schools as well as in nursing and medical schools in order to pursue their careers, often with the express purpose of being of service to their communities. Along with community health representatives and other community-based health workers, these Indigenous professionals, as critical observers of the system, have confronted barriers of racism and inequity, identified distinct health issues faced by Indigenous people in Canada, and worked to address systemic issues faced by all patients and health care workers. Such efforts have been complemented by those of Indigenous people who administer, analyze, teach, and research in faculties of medicine and nursing as well as in other areas, including community-based organizations. All remain significantly under-represented and yet considerably challenge the medical establishment and false assumptions about Indigenous people and their health that still by and large underlie health care.

Mainstream Canada overestimates the amount of state support for Indigenous and especially First Nations' health and underestimates the amount of state support for the universal health care enjoyed by Canadians and widely understood as a pillar of the Canadian identity. There is a deep structural racial segregation in health care, and it is at the root of the indifference with which Indigenous people are treated in health care institutions today: since Indigenous patients do not "really" belong, they do not deserve the same level of treatment as non-Indigenous patients, and their care is never quite as urgent, their needs never quite legitimate. The outrageousness of this inequality occasionally breaks through the fog of settler common sense, as it did in the case of Jordan's Principle. Jordan's Principle is named after Jordan River Anderson, a Cree child from Norway House, Manitoba, who was born in 1999 with a rare muscular disorder and required specialized care that could not be provided on reserve. Jordan spent more than two years at the HSC in Winnipeg before doctors decided he could return home to Norway House. However, provincial and federal governments, locked in a protracted fight over who was financially responsible for his home care, each refused to pay for his in-home care, and Jordan spent the rest of his life waiting, tragically dying at the HSC in 2005 still far away from his family home. Jordan's Principle dictates that the government of first contact with the child must fund the service so that jurisdictional disputes do not interfere with First Nations children accessing services that are available to other Canadian children.

Jordan's case made clear that First Nations children are frequently without services that they need and their care is often thwarted by complex jurisdictional politics, leaving children caught in the middle. While Jordan's Principle was unanimously passed in 2007 by the House of Commons, the federal government has implemented only a narrow interpretation of it, and was found by the Canadian Human Rights Tribunal to be racially discriminating against "165,000 First Nations children and their families for its failure to provide equitable services, including the proper implementation of Jordan's Principle." The tribunal has issued three sets of non-compliance orders, and from July to December 2017 more than 33,000 requests for support have been approved.[48] Currently, inequities in services are so common that the federal government has committed to a dedicated call centre to help families access the products, services, and supports they need under Jordan's Principle. For its part, the Manitoba legislature actually voted twice against ratifying Jordan's Principle before approving it in 2008.[49]

Who are the subjects born of these historical arrangements? Settlers committed to their superiority and to systems that endanger Indigenous life and Indigenous people who are imperilled at every turn. Why is it important to acknowledge that Brian Sinclair confronted these ideas, this knowledge, when he went to the HSC Winnipeg? We believe it is because this is an important first step in understanding how his life ended as it did. A different outcome would demand that we recognize and challenge fundamental structures of our society—ones based not simply on a benign inequality, or the poor behaviour of one person or a handful of them, but on an inequality that is built on the historical and continuing theft of resources and land, that is the air we all breathe. The final insult of colonization is that the myths of our settler society hold that ill health and early deaths of Indigenous people are their own fault, bearing no relation to the historical context of social, economic, and cultural oppression stemming from colonialism, white supremacy, and racism right here at home.

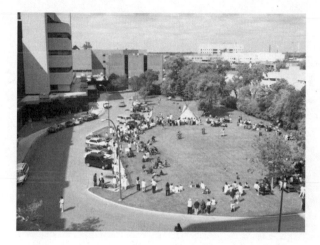

Figure 20.   A powwow held on the front lawn of the
Health Sciences Centre, 5 September 1997. Racism in
hospitals exists not in the absence of Indigenous people
and culture, but in their presence.

BRIAN SINCLAIR

3

THIS IS A STORY OF a city and a hospital, but more than that it is the story of a person, Brian Sinclair. In this chapter, we turn our focus to him. In particular, we explore how Sinclair's history illustrates some of the critical themes of twentieth- and twenty-first-century Indigenous history in Winnipeg, Manitoba, and Canada. We also show how the repeated misidentification of Sinclair in his final thirty-four hours waiting in the emergency room (ER) of Winnipeg's Health Sciences Centre hospital, and in the aftermath of his death reveals how structures of indifference born of colonialism and racism affect Indigenous people in the most fundamental and consequential of ways.

It is a truism that ordinary people's lives are not often recorded in the written archives upon which historians usually rely. This is certainly true for Indigenous people in North America, who historically have relied more on oral, material, and non-alphabetic means of recording information, and whose relationship to the colonial archive created from the sixteenth century onwards has been complicated, partial, and often contested. Our analysis here depends on twenty-first century colonial records available in libraries and online, namely newspapers and the records associated with the inquest into Brian Sinclair's death. The first phase of the inquest began in August 2013, lasted thirty-two days, and heard evidence from seventy-four witnesses. The judge decided that the second phase would be narrower in scope, against the urging of the Sinclair family and organizations who hoped that the inquest would document complex and deeply intersectional histories of racism, poverty, and unequal access to health care. While the scope of the inquest was initially broadly defined, and considered racism, poverty, health, and economic status as all relevant to the case, Judge Timothy Preston ruled that the scope of Phase II would focus on best practices for the ongoing training for frontline staff and that social determinants of health, such as race, poverty, and disability were not within the scope of the inquest.

Conducted in 2014, Phase II was completed in thirteen days; seven witnesses were staff of the Winnipeg Regional Health Authority, and of the seven, six would be called to testify about triage and how patients moved through the HSC ER. Only two witnesses addressed issues of stereotyping and racism.[1] As a result, almost all of the focus of Phase II was on sightlines within the ER, the triage process, delays in the ER, and staffing levels, even though these issues had posed no problems for the 150 people who received attention at the HSC ER on the same weekend Brian Sinclair died. The issues of stereotyping, false assumptions, and racism within the health care setting were reduced to just two witnesses whose evidence took less than one day. Because of the new, narrower focus on ER procedures, many of the recommendations in the inquest report have little or nothing to do with the death of Brian Sinclair, and the inquest evaded a prime opportunity to address and document issues of racism and colonialism in health care.

The limitations of this particular inquest were carefully and publicly noted at the time. For all its shortcomings, the Brian Sinclair inquest provided useful and important documentation of this Indigenous life and death. Certainly it is a substantial archive. Altogether, the consolidated transcripts from the two phases of the inquest run more than 4,500 pages in length, and Preston's report, issued in December 2014, is another 200 pages.[2] It is important to consider what the inquest did record and what it did not, what it included and what it excluded, and who participated and who felt compelled to withdraw. The documents produced by the inquest into Brian Sinclair's death comprise an archive that allows us to connect Sinclair's life, and the way it was seen, to the histories mapped in this book.

This archive only exists because of the terrible and wholly unnecessary way that Brian Sinclair's life ended. It is in no small part an archive of catastrophe and trauma. It is also an archive of resistance. In the days and weeks that followed his death, Sinclair's family and community successfully advocated for his death to be recognized, studied, and quite literally *seen* and acted on. In February of 2014, the Sinclair family explained that they had two objectives in pursuing an inquest: "to get the facts out" and "to have this inquest make recommendations for systematic changes to prevent similar tragedies to marginalized people like Brian Sinclair."[3]

In the pages of this archive of loss and resistance are some key details about Brian Sinclair's life that often go missing in the larger context. Esther Joyce Grant, Brian Sinclair's eldest sister, testified before the inquest in August of 2013 and provided biographical detail that ensured that her brother would not be misunderstood, neglected, and forgotten in the archive as he was in the hospital waiting room. The stories she shared told of a tidy, trustworthy younger brother with whom she had a special connection. Grant and Sinclair were part of a family of nine children born to Veronique Goosehead and Albert Sinclair. Goosehead had attended residential school. After completing Grade 11, she moved to Fort Alexander, an Anishinaabeg community in Treaty 1, now known as Sagkeeng

First Nation. There she met and married Albert Sinclair. The family was not recognized as status Indians under Canadian law and so lived off-reserve.[4] Like many Indigenous people in twentieth- and twenty-first-century Canada, the Sinclair family was wholly outside the ambit of rights and recognition that accompany Indian status. Scholars and activists have associated this exclusion with the particular predicaments faced by women under the sharply gendered terms of the Indian Act. Until 1985, the Indian Act legislated that women (and subsequently their children) lost status when they married non-status men.[5] And this is presumably what happened to Veronique Goosehead when she married Sinclair; their nine children were born without status.

In 1985, decades of activism from Indigenous women and legal challenges at multiple levels of government resulted in the passage of Bill C-31. This legislation removed some of the most egregiously sexist components from the Indian Act and provided a formula by which women who had been deleted from band lists upon marriage to non-status men, and their children, could apply for Indian status. Some of Sinclair's siblings were among the 114,412 people who by 2000 had gained their status based on Bill C-31 amendments.[6] Brian Sinclair, too, met the criteria to have his status restored through Bill C-31, as his sister noted during the inquest.[7] Yet Brian Sinclair's status was never restored, and whatever

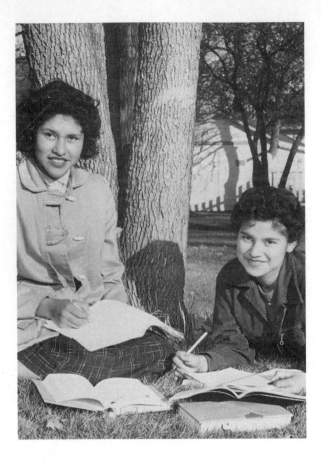

Figure 21. Schools perpetuated structures of indifference, teaching students that Indigenous people had little knowledge, history, or role in modern life. Here, Adeline Racette and Emma Bone, c. 1958, study outside the Assiniboia Residential School in Winnipeg's River Heights (1958–1973).

services he received, he did so as a resident of Manitoba and a citizen of Canada, not as a status Indian. His experience makes clear that much of the racialized logic of health care that we mapped in Chapter 2 remains in motion even when, as in this case, the person is not recognized as a status Indian.

Brian Sinclair lived with the complicated histories and experiences of many Indigenous people, including residential schooling and child apprehension and removal. As the circumstances leading up to his death make clear, Sinclair was racialized in very certain terms as a "Native" or "Aboriginal" person by those who encountered him, and he suffered fatally for that. As Chelsea Vowel has argued, mainstream Canadian views chronically underestimate the taxes Indigenous people pay and overestimate the resources they receive in terms of education, health, and other social services.[8] In any case, the benefits and services that Sinclair was entitled to as a non-status Indigenous person were mainly the same ones that other Manitobans take for granted. Like countless other Indigenous people, especially visibly Indigenous ones, Brian Sinclair lived with difficult histories and ongoing presents and received little of the resources associated with Indigenous or treaty rights.

The history of the Sinclair family also suggests some of the contours of Indigenous wage labour and modernity. Albert Sinclair was a commercial fisherman and a logger, remembered by his eldest daughter as "a very hardworking man." Brian was born in 1963, and when he was a toddler the family moved to Powerview, just south of Sagkeeng First Nation, about 120 kilometres northeast of Winnipeg.[9] Powerview and the adjacent community of Pine Falls formed a site of twentieth-century resource development and planning, a place whose commerce depended on hydroelectric development and forestry. Built along the Winnipeg River, the town was created in the mid-1920s when a newsprint mill attracted a large workforce to the area.

The land on which the mill town was built was acquired by entrepreneur John D. McArthur through a complicated process negotiated by the Department of Indian Affairs and not in the best interests of First Nations. The 1920s were the tail end of a huge theft of reserve land through the mechanisms of leasing and surrender: more than a hundred surrenders of prairie reserve land were obtained by Canada between the 1890s and 1930s. Between 1896 and 1911 alone, a remarkable 21 percent of lands reserved to First Nations in Manitoba, Alberta, and Saskatchewan were surrendered.[10] These numbers reflected changes to Department of Indian Affairs policy that facilitated the process by which First Nations could legally be stripped of their rights to reserve lands. "Surrender" was one of the main ways that this occurred. Usually, a meeting of male band members over twenty-one was held, and if the support of a majority was obtained, the surrender was approved, and the lands and resources were lost to the First Nation. It is not hard to find examples where such deals favoured the interests of settlers and industrial capitalists and resulted in hardship for First Nations. It is also not hard to find examples where the surrender process was baldly manipulated. The loss of the St. Peter's Reserve, a prosperous agricultural community in southern Manitoba, in 1907 is particularly revealing of the ways "surrender" could be and was used.[11]

Pine Falls grew substantially with the construction of the nearby hydro-power generating station in 1952. In 1976, the mill at Powerview–Pine Falls produced 480 tonnes of newsprint a day and was the only newspaper-making facility in the Canadian prairies.[12] This snippet of history is a window into the story of Indigenous people's wage work in postwar Manitoba and Canada, well beyond the heyday of the fur trade, a neglected story that historians have told only in bits and pieces.[13] Such accounts are unfamiliar to many, and are a needed corrective to the erroneous and dismissive stereotypes of Indigenous people and mainstream histories of Indigenous-land relations.

Stories of child welfare, and more particularly child removal and apprehension, are another critical part of Indigenous people's history within modern Canada and other settler societies. As residential schooling declined in the years following the Second

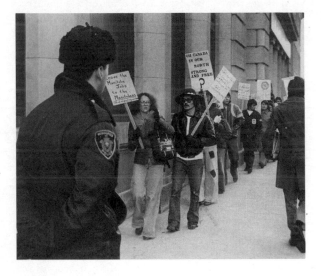

Figure 22. In 1979, the Manitoba Metis Federation picketed the federal government office responsible for employment and unemployment in downtown Winnipeg, demanding more and better-paid work. Note the watchful City of Winnipeg police officer.

World War, practices of child removal into state care for fostering and adoption increased. What became known as the Sixties Scoop actually began earlier and lasted longer. By the 1970s, 60 percent of the children in care in Manitoba were Indigenous.[14] Brian Sinclair and his brothers were some of those children. In the early 1970s, the Sinclair family moved to Winnipeg's North End and entered a difficult stretch. The younger children began to hang out with kids who used solvents; Albert and Veronique separated, and at times struggled with alcohol. At some point, "Children's Aid came and got" the younger children. This intervention was not permanent. Albert Sinclair got his kids back, and he and Brian remained close.[15] This story of Indigenous families and child welfare systems is not the one we generally associate with the Sixties Scoop, which more often aimed for the permanent adoption of children into non-Indigenous families. But the story of children being removed and placed into local foster care is all too familiar.[16]

Like many Indigenous people in twentieth- and twenty-first-century Canada, Brian Sinclair was poor and, as a result, at times housing insecure and vulnerable. As an adult, Brian and his brothers Russell and Bradley lived in a rooming house on William Avenue. The arrangement fell apart when their landlady sold the house.[17] In January 2007, when Brian Sinclair was forty-three, he was locked out of his rooming house in the Winnipeg winter and suffered from hypothermia and frostbite so severe that both of his legs had to be amputated above the knee. That January included nineteen days in which the thermometer dropped to –20°C or below, seven of those below –30°C. While Sinclair was being treated for his amputation at the HSC, a doctor's recommendation set in motion a series of steps that concluded with Sinclair's physician issuing a "certificate of incapacity" and forwarding it for review by the province's chief psychiatrist, under the province's Mental Health Act. Sinclair was then appointed a Public Trustee of the Office of the Public Guardian and Trustee of Manitoba, an office that, among other things, "administers estates and makes personal decisions on behalf of mentally incompetent adults or vulnerable adults who are not mentally capable of making decisions independently."[18] From 2007 onwards, Sinclair was visibly disabled and used a wheelchair. He was also subject to a particular and highly personalized mode of state control, one secured through provincial legislation and medicalized authority.

The relatives, community resources, and service providers who spoke at the inquest into Brian Sinclair's death inadvertently provide a kind of counter-narrative to the structures of indifference that he encountered throughout his life and, finally, in the HSC ER in September of 2008. In their recall of Sinclair's upbringing, his character and how he spent his days, and the support he received, witnesses provided evidence of a life lived within a community. Whatever his challenges were, Sinclair was neither without resources nor alone. He was close to his two brothers and remained in touch with his sister in Vancouver, though Sinclair did not tell her about the loss of his legs. In these years, Sinclair lived at the Quest Inn and Assisted Living Centre. This is a downtown motel refurbished by the Winnipeg Regional Health Authority that, since 2002, has provided "medical needs accommodation" and meals for short and, as in Sinclair's case, long stays.[19] At the Quest Inn, Sinclair received assisted living services and maintained close relationships with a number of his caregivers. In their testimony to the inquest, support and home-care workers who had worked closely with Sinclair in the last year and a half of his life spoke of an orderly and independent man who struggled with communication issues, was critical of disruptive neighbours, and could resent intrusions into his life and routine. Sinclair was a regular visitor to at least two missions: the Lighthouse and, especially, Siloam Mission, a self-described "Christian humanitarian organization" that, since 1987, has provided services and resources for poor and homeless people in downtown Winnipeg.[20] The minister of the Lighthouse described Sinclair as "the epitome of patience," a person who did not complain even when "there were things he could complain about."[21] Sinclair spent much of his days at Siloam, in part for the "camaraderie" and

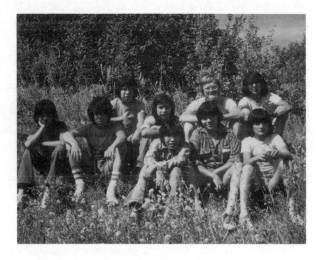

Figure 23. This photo shows Brian Sinclair at a
semi-wilderness camp called Camp Neecheewam,
located north of Winnipeg in the Interlake region, in
1977. Brian is fourteen in the photo. He is fourth from
the left, sitting beside teacher Karl Gomph.

to stay in touch with his brothers, friends, and what homecare worker Darwin Ironstand called "his social network."[22] Sinclair also volunteered at Siloam, and he spoke of this work with pride.[23] Within the roughly two-kilometre familiar geography that included his home at the Quest Inn and his volunteer work and social connections at the Siloam Mission, Sinclair and his brothers were well known (see Figure 24). "Everybody knew these fellows, the community, the downtown community in that area, everybody knows everybody, or many people know everybody," explained one witness.[24]

As a double-amputee with an indwelling catheter, Sinclair had distinct medical needs. He also lived with a set of communication and perhaps cognitive issues, ones that received a great deal of attention but not a lot of diagnostic clarity during the inquest that examined his death. In the last years of his life, Sinclair received services funded through provincial programs and delivered within his familiar geography: thrice daily homecare visits, twice weekly visits from an "integrated service worker," weekly home support for laundry, and a visit from a nurse every other week.[25] This was supplemented by speech therapy, contact with a nurse practitioner at Siloam Mission and physicians at the Health Action Centre, and occasional trips to the HSC. Between 2003 and 2008, Brian Sinclair visited the HSC a total of thirty-one times, or an average of about six times a year.[26]

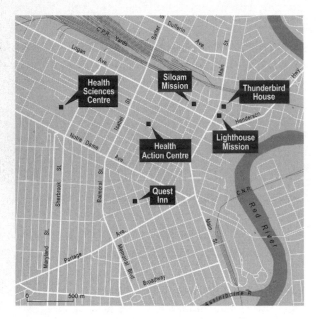

Figure 24.   This map highlights the area in Winnipeg where Brian Sinclair spent much of his time during the last few years of his life.

The way Sinclair died, and how his death was understood, speak to the fatal consequences that ordinary racism has on Indigenous lives. These social relations were at play in a context where Indigenous people were present in robust numbers. Certainly, this was the case during Sinclair's last days spent in the HSC ER waiting room. There he was one of what one of the nurses described as a "vast majority" of Indigenous patients.[27] Enduring patterns of racialized work that developed in late nineteenth- and twentieth-century Canada and persisted into the new millennium meant that labour in hospitals like the HSC is unlikely to have been significantly Indigenous, but some of Sinclair's brief interactions during that time at the HSC were with an Indigenous security guard.[28] As Leslie Spillett, then the executive director of Ka Ni Kanichihk, explained in her address before the first phase of the inquest, Sinclair had a "lethal intersection" of social identities.[29] Sinclair was not simply Indigenous, but middle-aged and visibly disabled. We are best equipped to understand his experiences, and the ways that he was seen and not seen, when we take an intersectional approach that registers how identities and structures—in this case race, indigeneity, ability, gender, and social class—co-produce experience, and, for Brian Sinclair, death.

The structures of indifference that Sinclair encountered during those thirty-four hours converged around a set of images associated with Indigenous men. Scholars Kim Anderson and Robert Innes have argued that the conditions of Indigenous men are in many ways similar to those of Indigenous women, "but these conditions have not really been acknowledged beyond news reports of their criminal behavior."[30] In media reporting and inquiries into Sinclair's death two particular misidentifications came up again and again: homelessness and drunkenness. In print and broadcast media, local and national, Sinclair was routinely described as homeless. He was described this way in the days following his death in 2008, and years later.[31] The information available in public records suggests that Sinclair had been housing insecure during points of his life, but in the last year and a half of his life he had a permanent residence at the Quest Inn. The repeated labelling of Sinclair as homeless suggests the figurative work that the term can perform, working not as a description of a person's housing, but as shorthand for a certain presentation of poverty, one that in many Canadian cities, and certainly in Winnipeg, is racialized as Indigenous. We can acknowledge that Indigenous people are over-represented in the homeless population of Winnipeg, and Canada as a whole,[32] while also recognizing the discursive work performed by the casual connection between Indigeneity, disability, and homelessness.

In Sinclair's case, the repeated description of him as homeless rendered a brittle and inaccurate stock image that robbed him of his real and complex humanity. Labelling Sinclair as homeless misrepresented him and also worked to render invisible people in his life and their work with and care for Sinclair. At the inquest, people who had cared for Sinclair pushed back against this description. One of Sinclair's home-care workers explained that "it was very upsetting to the people who worked with him that he was described as homeless because they cared for him an awful lot and they felt that that should be recognized."[33]

A corollary to the misrecognition of Brian Sinclair as homeless was the presumption that he was in the waiting room of the HSC ER not because he had urgent medical needs, but because he simply needed somewhere to go, to stay warm, or to pass the time. Winnipeg winters are long and cold, but Brian Sinclair spent his final hours in the HSC ER in September and the weather was mild and dry, with a high of 21°C and a low of 7.3°C.[34] Nor does Sinclair appear to have lacked for places to go to pass the time, locate resources, or find company. Those who spoke knowledgeably of Sinclair's last year and a half made clear that he routinely spent his days away from his residence, visiting and volunteering at Siloam Mission, attending to medical and other appointments, and shopping. Sinclair was poor, but he was not without spending money. At the time of his death Brian Sinclair had approximately $5,000 in the bank.[35]

In his thirty-four hours in the HSC emergency room, Sinclair was also repeatedly misrecognized as drunk. There is a long and remarkably tenacious assumption that Indigenous people, across North America and beyond, are somehow predisposed to alcoholism and disproportionately likely to be problem drinkers. The trope of the "drunken Indian," explain Roxanne Dunbar-Ortiz and Dina Gilio-Whitaker, is intractable, damaging, and deeply woven into American social narratives, popular and scholarly.[36] Specifically examining the Canadian context, Vowel notes that widely available scholarship has helped to debunk some of these stereotypes or at least render them less powerful.[37] But the case of Brian Sinclair reaffirms her point that assumptions about Indigenous people and drunkenness persist in Canadian society and popular culture, and do real damage to Indigenous lives.

The evidence presented to the inquest makes clear exactly how far Brian Sinclair's life was from these damaging scripts. It is not that Sinclair had no history of substance use or contact with the law, something that is not surprising given practices of policing and patterns of incarceration in Winnipeg. Testimony before the inquest revealed that Sinclair had been locked up six times under the Intoxicated Persons Detention Act, which allows police to detain an individual without criminal charges. The Winnipeg police officer who testified at the inquest agreed with the Sinclair family lawyer that "although Mr. Sinclair had struggled with substance abuse for most of his life, he had relatively minimal exposure to the justice system."[38] These incidents were also far in Sinclair's past: all but one occurred between 1993 and 2002.[39] Of Sinclair's thirty-one trips to the HSC ER between 2003 and 2008, only one in 2006 was related to substance use. Otherwise, Sinclair visited the ER for treatment of seizures, trauma, urinary tract complaints, and other medical issues.[40]

In testimony before the inquest, these damaging misrecognitions came up again and again and were used to explain, retroactively predict, or otherwise naturalize Sinclair's death and reinforce the idea that he was in the HSC ER for something other than a genuine and pressing medical need. After his review of Sinclair's medical history, neuropathologist Mark Del Bigio wrote an email to the province's medical examiner and CEO of the Winnipeg Regional Health Authority in which he explained that Sinclair's demise was a direct result of substance use, and his own fault. "We should not lose sight of the fact that the man's problems were self-inflicted," wrote Del Bigio in June 2009.[41] By the time of the inquest some three years later, Del Bigio and forensic pathologist Thambirajah Balachandra, then Chief Medical Examiner for Manitoba, were both careful to recognize that Sinclair had died from a bladder infection that could have been easily treated with a catheter change and antibiotics, to acknowledge that Sinclair was not homeless, and to agree that there was no evidence to suggest that Sinclair was in any way intoxicated, not that intoxication could have explained his medical issues or death in any event.[42] Their evidence instead focused on neurological and medical co-morbidities discovered through the processes of medical examination. At the inquest, officials argued that these "co-morbidities prevented Mr. Sinclair from 'fighting harder' to stay alive," as the judge summarized in his final report released late in 2014.[43]

This representation of Sinclair as a "medically vulnerable" person with serious co-morbidities worked to reframe and make palatable the idea that he was somehow already dying or responsible for his own predictable death and make this story fit with the evidence that he had died for want of basic medical attention in a hospital waiting room. What was presented in much of the testimony before the inquest and in the final report became a nuanced variation on what Razack describes as the "logic of the 'vanishing Indian,' the construct, that is, of a pathologically fragile individual belonging to a race for whom death is always imminent."[44] As in the inquests into the death by suicide of two Indigenous teenage girls in the Manitoba Youth Centre studied by Mandi Gray, the death of Brian Sinclair was framed and managed as the primary result of "individual pathology."[45] It was also framed as the tragic outcome of a stressed, understaffed, and imperfectly organized ER.

Putting emphasis on Sinclair as an individual and on the organization of the HSC ER gestures to but ultimately avoids reckoning with the fact that Sinclair's life was lost because he received no care in the very place he was told to expect it, that he was allowed to sicken and die over a thirty-four-hour period and in plain view of staff and patients. Brian Sinclair died because the hospital failed to care for him, and because he lived in a world that was carefully calibrated to produce Indigenous suffering and then both rationalize and be indifferent to it. This is but one example of a structure of indifference that is both pervasive and deadly. It is on full display in the inquest into the deaths of seven Anishinaabeg teenagers in Thunder Bay, Ontario, between 2000 and 2011, so evocatively analyzed by journalist Tanya Talaga.[46] Examples like these, of what Razack describes as the "casual inhumanity" and "deep disregard for Indigenous life,"[47] are threaded throughout modern Canadian life and are found *everywhere*.

CONCLUSION

IT HAS BEEN TEN YEARS since Brian Sinclair died in the waiting room of Winnipeg's Health Sciences Centre ER. In that time, Sinclair's family and the Indigenous community in Winnipeg, Manitoba, and Canada have worked to ensure that his death would not be forgotten and have fought for necessary reforms. The inquest into Sinclair's death is evidence of their advocacy and persistence and also of the limits of these sorts of inquiries. As in the inquests into the deaths of two young Anishinaabeg men in Kashechewan studied by Carmela Murdocca, we might read the inquest into Brian Sinclair's death as a moment when the colonial state strains "to find ways to capture evidence and demarcate the boundaries of legal, governmental and political responsibility and failure."[1]

Throughout the inquest, the official narrative was that Sinclair's death was a "one-off." In his opening address, the Winnipeg Regional Health Authority's lawyer explained that "a perfect storm occurred whereby the weaknesses and deficiencies in the system and the staff employed at the HSC, collectively, were causative of this tragedy."[2] Judge Timothy Preston, in his final report, expressed his support for this metaphor.[3] The metaphor of the storm works to associate the events of September 2008 with the natural world, a proverbial act of God, well outside human causality. Two key corollaries accompany the "perfect storm" argument. The first is that no single person could be "responsible" for what happened, and, simultaneously, that Sinclair himself, soft-spoken, hard to understand, and with cognitive challenges, also contributed to this perfect storm. His very presence and being were, in part, to blame; that is, he just simply should not have been there, or perhaps simply should not have been at all. The second corollary is the assertion that this *coincidental* mass collision of multiple errors could have happened to anyone. Indeed, in his testimony, the Chief Medical Examiner of Manitoba, Thambirajah Balachandra, argued that "even if Snow White came in the wheelchair on that day, this situation, she would have died."[4] The gendered, racialized, and physical dimensions of the choice of metaphor here are not incidental.

Within the logic of the "perfect storm," the systems and processes of the hospital came under scrutiny rather than the ways Sinclair was repeatedly misrecognized by medical and support staff, and how misrecognitions justified the many times that Sinclair

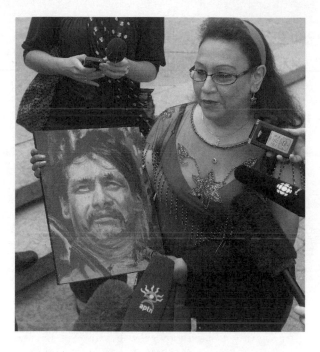

Figure 25. Brian Sinclair's sister holds a portrait of him by artist Gord Hagman outside the courthouse, 6 August 2013. The family asked to display the portrait in the courtroom during the inquest as a reminder that he was a loved human being, not just a headline. The judge denied their request (a copy was instead submitted as Exhibit 22).

was ignored or dismissed. Behind these misrecognitions is the belief that Sinclair was not really in need of or deserving of care, that his presence in a hospital was at its core illegitimate and things were bound to go awry. And yet Sinclair's death was linked instead primarily to multiple failures in the policies and procedures of processing patients in the ER.

The system of triage was examined with particular care. Normally in ER protocol a triage nurse obtains details about a medical complaint and decides how to prioritize the patient and where they are to go by talking to and visually examining the patient and taking vital signs. The triage process identifies urgent, life-threatening conditions, initiates tests and treatments, and determines the most appropriate treatment site or area for patients. It involves the ongoing assessment of waiting room patients and the relaying of information to patients and families regarding services, expected care, and wait times. The argument here follows that because Sinclair was not triaged and registered as a patient of the ER, he was not treated. Because the cause of his death was attributed to his not being triaged, it followed that fixing the triage process would prevent this kind of tragedy from happening in the future.

Triage and the "perfect storm" became red herrings in Sinclair's case, ways of diverting attention from issues of racism and colonialism. Triage is referred to about 350 times in the final report of the inquest; race or racism is mentioned only thirteen times. The report represents triage as being outside of racism (which is inherently another sorting project), as a scientific, colour-blind process that assesses bodies devoid of cultural, social, intellectual, and racial meaning. For example, Balachandra testified that he had "never come across a nurse, attendant, doctor, anybody discriminating on the basis of anything other than the disease itself," insisting that staff put aside their own opinions.[5] This sentiment was repeated by a nurse who had been on duty when Sinclair spent his last thirty-four hours in the waiting room. She explained that "it wouldn't matter what race he was."[6] In their testimony before the inquest, many witnesses indicated that the idea that racism might have played into the events of September 2008 was absurd, even unimaginable. They suggested that racism was an impossibility, since the majority of HSC patients were Indigenous—as if racism was more or less an act of discrimination or bigotry against a distinct and literal minority. The more layered and complex framings of structural racism and its effects in the particular context of Winnipeg that witnesses and participants like Leslie Spillett provided, ultimately, had a modest role in the inquest and an even smaller one in the report.

Sinclair was indeed subject to a very real process of triage. He was, in fact, triaged in a way that is implicit in our health care system in highly racialized practices that are systemic, structural, primary, and invisible. Here we want to centre Indigenous people in an understanding of the everyday ways triage is racialized in Manitoba, in Canada, and in other settler colonial contexts. Drawing on the work of scholars in Indigenous history and other fields, we can put the HSC ER in a broader historical context: we know that in settler colonial contexts, the lives of Indigenous people are valued less than those of non-Indigenous people, and in these contexts Indigenous health declines and inequities develop. We also know that, historically and still today, Canadian governments believe health care for Indigenous people should always be cheaper than it is for others and that health care is not only, and sometimes not even primarily, about biomedicine—it is also about assimilation and integration into the Canadian nation state and the annulment of treaty rights and responsibilities, as well as erasure of Indigenous autonomy, identity, and ways of life.

A body of work on racism in health care confirms that Indigenous patients are often concerned that they will be treated differently, which leads them to strategize how they might deal with anticipated racism before they go to the hospital or even to avoid care if possible.[7] We need to see health care as a terrain of racism and colonialism, one that costs lives. As Metis physician and researcher Janet Smylie explains, the impact of racism in health care is neither abstract nor subtle: "people are dying unnecessarily or experiencing disability."[8] There is good reason that health plays a significant role in the TRC's Calls to Action. Calls 18 through 24 address the role that health care has played in colonialism and call on federal and provincial governments to make serious and far-reaching changes: to "acknowledge that the current state of Aboriginal health in Canada is a direct result of previous Canadian government policies"; to work towards identifying and closing the gaps in health outcomes between Indigenous and non-Indigenous people; to recognize the distinct health needs of Metis, Inuit, and off-reserve Indigenous people; for the federal government to fund Aboriginal healing centres; to recognize the value of indigenous healing practices; to increase the number of Indigenous professionals in health care and provide "cultural competency training for all health care professionals"; and for medical and nursing schools to require students to take a wide-ranging course on Indigenous health issues.[9] Some of these are directions that have been taken in and around Winnipeg for some time. As the photographs of the Native Medical Interpreters Course graduates in 1986 (Figure 19) and of the powwow held on HSC grounds in 1997 (Figure 20) included in Chapter 2 make clear, efforts to address the particular health care needs of Indigenous people and to integrate aspects of Indigenous culture into health care have been underway for some time; they did not prevent Brian Sinclair from dying in the HSC emergency department from a very treatable infection. The TRC's Calls to Action make clear that more robust and thorough-going change is required—change, that is, to the structure of health care, and of Canada.

The structures of indifference that Sinclair encountered at the HSC ER had lethal consequences. They were not natural, or accidental, or without precedence. The structures of indifference continued in the inquest that investigated what went wrong in the ER over those thirty-four hours. In a way, the Brian Sinclair inquest is characteristic of the ways Canadian hospitals address racism. If patients are racialized as Indigenous by appearance, assumptions will be made not only about their state of health but also about whether or not they belong in a hospital or even if they deserve care at all. This can lead directly to under-treatment of Indigenous people in the health care system. Tania Dick, a nurse from the Dzawada'enuxw First Nation of Kingcome Inlet and president of the Association of Registered Nurses of British Columbia, agrees: "My family has a Brian Sinclair story. . . . I have the privilege and opportunity with the role I'm in to travel throughout different communities and everywhere I went they had a Brian Sinclair story."[10] In this context, the experiences of Brian Sinclair and those of other Indigenous families with their own "Brian Sinclair story" are not anomalous, but reflect the ways that Indigenous people have been constructed as being beyond or outside health care, often with tragic results for Indigenous people who do find themselves in hospitals.

The story of Brian Sinclair makes the most sense to us when we locate it within the histories of Winnipeg, Manitoba, Canada, and racialized medicine. Seen in this way, what happened to him in the waiting room of the HSC ER was one chapter in the revealing and devastating histories of dispossession and colonial violence. The hospital itself, including its ER, is part of a system that privileges some while robbing others of their health and well-being and even their lives. As discussed in Chapter 2, the *longue durée* history of the HSC involves the transfer of Indigenous lands as well as Indigenous funds and labour through many hands over a period that was not so long ago. More recently, this hospital, like those throughout western Canada, was a centre for the training of doctors and nurses who went out to work in segregated hospitals—both Indian and white. Hospitals occupy a special place in histories of modern Canadian segregation. These segregationist practices were contested and remade by the social changes of the postwar era, ones that brought Sinclair's family, among many other Indigenous families, to cities like Winnipeg. The system of formally segregated health care studied by Maureen Lux and others was revised in the 1980s and 1990s,[11] but the extent to which hospitals like the HSC remain problematic spaces for people like Sinclair makes clear how these histories continue to reverberate through the present.

What happens to Indigenous people across Canada in hospital waiting rooms suggests that the hospital continues to be a particular site of colonial history and contest. It is not hard to find versions of what happened to Brian Sinclair across Canada. In the summer of 2017 a forty-three-year-old Mi'kmaq woman whose health card had been stolen left Montreal's McGill University Health Centre after being told that she would need to pay $1,400 to see a doctor. She died, alone and untreated, a month later. In the fall of that month, a fifty-five-year-old Stó:lō woman with multiple fractures was twice sent away from a hospital in Chilliwack, British Columbia.[12]

Brian Sinclair's story, like all the Brian Sinclair stories from hospitals across Canada, shows how this country's institutions have failed and continue to fail Indigenous people by undermining and devaluing Indigenous life. During the writing of this book, we have been motivated by an intensely violent, but also creative and productive moment, in Winnipeg and beyond. It is a moment of heightened visibility of anti-Indigenous racism, injustice, and marginalization—a moment when the politics of colonization and resistance, Indigenous sovereignty, and subordination have become topics in mainstream media—regardless of how well or badly covered. Anti-Indigenous racism, it seems, is something that everyone has an opinion about.

In 2017 and 2018 court cases and inquests resulting from three Indigenous deaths became a focus for a politics of Indigenous and ally activism. The first is the trial of Raymond Cormier, who was charged with second-degree murder in the death of fifteen-year-old Tina Fontaine. Like Brian Sinclair, Tina was from Sagkeeng First Nation and was embroiled in systems of care that failed to protect her. Her body was found in the Red River in August 2014, wrapped in a duvet weighted with rocks. Fontaine's death became a focal point of discussions about gendered racism and renewed calls for a national inquiry into missing and murdered Indigenous women. This inquiry is now under way, in the process of holding community hearings and gathering statements. Shortly after Fontaine's body was found in the river, Kyle Kematch and Bernadette Smith, both family members of missing Indigenous women, came together to start Drag the Red—a community-based, volunteer-led initiative to search the bottom of the Red River for traces of other missing and murdered Indigenous people.

Despite what was by all accounts a serious police investigation, Cormier was found not guilty in February 2018. The broad strokes of the story itself are all too familiar. Fontaine was supposed to be under the care of Manitoba's Child and Family Services, then so under-resourced that it housed foster children in downtown Winnipeg hotels—a deplorable practice that loosened community ties and increased vulnerability of youth already in difficult circumstances. Police knew that Fontaine was in trouble and yet failed to protect her on multiple occasions, and no one was directly held responsible for these failures. Other common statistics provide some context for the case. According to the Interim Report of the National Inquiry into Missing and Murdered Indigenous Women and Girls, "Indigenous women experience intimate partner violence more frequently and more severely than do non-Indigenous women. Indigenous women are roughly seven times more likely than non-Indigenous women to be murdered by serial killers ... [and] Indigenous women are physically assaulted, sexually assaulted, or robbed almost three times as often as non-Indigenous women. . . . Simply being Indigenous and female is a risk."[13]

As we write this, another death of an Indigenous person in custody or care in Winnipeg is being examined at the inquest of twenty-six-year-old Errol Greene, who died of internal bleeding in 2016 after having two seizures at the Winnipeg Remand Centre, a pre-trial detention centre.

So far the inquest has pointed to clear issues of policy implicated in his death: Greene's medications were denied to him as a matter of prison policy, even

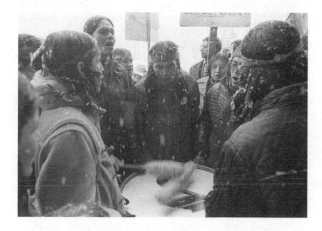

Figure 26. Modes of urban Indigenous protest have a long history. This drum group was part of an October 1972 protest by about 300 "Indians and Metis" who marched in the snow from the North End to the Manitoba Legislature, where Metis scholar and activist Howard Adams and other Indigenous leaders addressed the crowd.

after he had explained that he needed them and filled out two request forms. Greene was handcuffed and shackled during his seizures.[14] Yet such policies cannot be divorced from the larger context that Indigenous people are radically over-represented in Canadian jails. The numbers are higher in western Canada, and certainly Winnipeg's Remand Centre has a particular history to account for: Greene was one of five people who died there in 2016 alone.[15] The repeated indifference and lack of empathy Greene faced is characteristic of Indigenous deaths in custody, whether in jail or other institutions including schools, hospitals, and child welfare settings. These failings have been countered by the remarkable persistence and brave advocacy of Greene's widow and cellmate, who have continued to speak out and work with community activists to ensure that Greene's death be acknowledged and investigated.

The constant spectre of Indigenous death and the unwillingness of institutions to hold anything or anyone accountable (other than the deceased) are also apparent in the acquittal of Gerald Stanley in the shooting death of twenty-two-year-old Colten Boushie. The young Cree man was killed by a single bullet to the back of his head from a handgun fired by Stanley. On 9 August 2016, Colten Boushie and four friends drove onto a farm belonging to Gerald Stanley; Stanley and his son believed that they were there to steal. There was no evidence that Boushie ever got out of the car before being shot. The defence's line of argument was that Stanley's gun went off accidentally and that he never pulled the trigger, though expert testimony determined that was highly unlikely. As Cree scholars Gina Starblanket and Dallas Hunt have argued, the sequence of events that led to and surround the trial are "intimately tied to the histories of present-day settlement in the country currently called Canada" and the violence and dispossession that underpin it.[16] At the end of the trial, jurors were given three choices: second-degree murder, manslaughter, or acquittal. While second-degree murder was difficult to prove, at the very least, the charge of manslaughter—a dangerous act that causes death but without the intent to kill—would have been reasonable in this case. Jurors instead chose to acquit the defendant; something that happens in a mere 3 percent of Canadian murder trials overall. The jury is not permitted to discuss their proceedings, so we will never know the reasoning behind their decision. What we do know is a little of how the jury was chosen. In this case, the defence used peremptory challenges during the jury selection to eliminate all visibly Indigenous people from the jury, and the result was an apparently all-white jury in a part of Canada with a significant Indigenous population. What we know about the community in which the trial occurred can be gleaned from local media reports and, especially, the outpouring on social media of fear and blame stoked by racism and segregation. Meanwhile, Boushie's family and most Indigenous leaders and commentators urged peaceful responses aimed at reframing the narrative, articulating Colten's humanity, and addressing root issues. These are some of the concerns that are driving a cluster of federal initiatives and reforms, including a bill that would amend the Criminal Code with reference to jury selection.[17]

The flame of ordinary and banal Canadian racism has been fanned by the Stanley trial, and there has been a troubling backlash against Indigenous people, especially on social media. Some have received threatening emails or notes after speaking out about the verdict, and at least one Indigenous media website was suspiciously hacked after it posted a searing commentary about racism in the trial written by Salish journalist Robert Jago.[18] As Robert Innes notes, the fact that no charges for hate speech were laid when Indigenous lives were threatened in response to online discussions of this case is a further example of how anti-Indigenous racism in modern Canada is seen as more or less acceptable.[19]

History is about the past, but we research, write, and teach history in a political and social present that is neither independent of nor unconnected to it. September 2018 marks the ten-year anniversary of Brian Sinclair's death, and the connections between the past and the present are brought home to us in clear and urgent ways. The stories of Brian Sinclair, Tina Fontaine, Colten Boushie, and Errol Greene are all different. But theirs are all stories of Indigenous deaths and of the ways that settler institutions have both produced and failed to respond to these deaths, in effect normalizing them. In the past months, people across Canada have set up camps; held marches, public talks, and symposia; and organized social media campaigns like those for #JusticeforColten, #JusticeforErrol, and #LoveforTina. The untimely, difficult deaths of all of these Indigenous people were produced by histories of colonialism, of segregation, and of institutions, whether hospitals, jails, or foster care. These deaths were determined by the past and show the interlocking work of gender, race, Indigeneity, and age. They remind us that the past is far from over, and that we need to look it squarely in the eye if we are to make sense of the ways that Indigenous lives like that of Brian Sinclair—and like those of Fontaine, Greene, and Boushie—continue to be lost in a Canada that never wanted them in the first place and was predicated, in no small measure, on their disappearance. We likewise need to look at this history if we are to understand how the trials, inquests, and inquiries into Indigenous deaths work to simultaneously document and disavow the ways that racism and colonialism produce, and then effectively condone, the loss of Indigenous life.

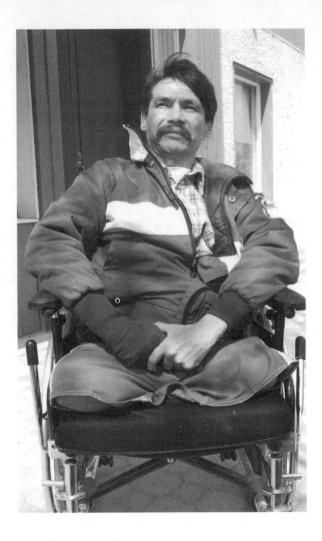

Figure 27. Brian Sinclair, 2008.

ACKNOWLEDGEMENTS

WHEN BRIAN SINCLAIR DIED IN September 2008, now already ten years ago, there was a widespread sense that a terribly unjust yet recurring and almost predictable tragedy had occurred. An accompanying sense of concern, sadness, hopelessness, and anger unfolded as we learned more and more details of how he died, and especially as the inquest into his death turned away from critically examining racism. This sense of inevitability comes from the structures of indifference that surround us, while our anger is a reminder that things can and should be different. At the release of the report of the inquest into the death of Brian Sinclair in December 2014, Brian's cousin Robert Sinclair stated: "This is not just a story about a bad triage system. It is a story about failing to show care and compassion for human beings based on assumptions about who they are. . . . As long as stereotyping still exists in our health care system, and as long as our health care, government and judicial institutions refuse to acknowledge or tackle the problem, we cannot say that we have succeeded. We cannot say that Brian Sinclair's death was not in vain."

In the wake of his death, Sinclair's family and Indigenous and other social justice organizations in Winnipeg and Manitoba have continued to challenge structural indifference and assert that Brian Sinclair deserved better. They told us to critically examine and address, rather than ignore and deny, how racism structures our experiences in life and in death. As historians and writers, we are indebted to their persistence and participation, especially at what must have been an extraordinarily difficult time and in circumstances framed only to marginalize them. The archive of the inquest documents their determination and willingness to speak truth to power.

We are also indebted to the work of the Brian Sinclair Working Group (BSWG). A large and shifting group of health and legal professionals, academics, and other leaders, the BSWG met many times in person and on the phone, and these conversations foregrounded the book in many ways. Special thanks go to Emily Hill, Barry Lavallee, Linda Diffey, Leslie Spillett, Brenda Gunn, Christa Big Canoe, and many others who engaged with the work of the BSWG and encouraged and supported the kind of rigorous public attention that the case merited.

Critical engagement with the book by audiences with a wide range of experience and expertise has immeasurably influenced it. Parts have been presented at: the Native American and Indigenous Studies Association annual conference; "Systemic Racism: Brian Sinclair's Story," an event hosted at the University of Manitoba Health Sciences Campus by Community Health Sciences, Max Rady College of Medicine, and Ongomiizwin-Education; the Faculty of Native Studies at the University of Alberta; and the Manitoba-Ontario-Minnesota-Saskatchewan History of Medicine Conference at the University of Winnipeg. We would like to thank the anonymous reviewers, who generously and constructively engaged with the book. Both readers graciously and with alacrity offered helpful suggestions and thoughtful responses that ultimately strengthened our book. The University of Winnipeg Indigenous Research Scholar Award helped to make this book possible.

Thanks to Jill McConkey for her reflection on and engagement with our writing on Sinclair and racism in health care. Her persistence made the book possible. Jill and Glenn Bergen at the University of Manitoba Press found a way to make the release of this book coincide with the tenth anniversary of Sinclair's death, which meant devising and keeping to a strict schedule.

A number of individuals have provided assistance at different junctures. Bella Malo, née Guimond (Pine Falls Health Complex), provided background information about the town of Powerview-Pine Falls, as well as photos of the hospital. Thanks to Niigaan Sinclair for some last-minute and appreciated help. We would also like to thank archivists and other staff Joanna Munholland (Sam Waller Museum), Tanya Wiegand (Health Sciences Centre Museum and Archives), Linda Eddy (University of Manitoba Archives and Special Collections), Karine Vinette (McCord Museum), and staff at Library and Archives Canada. We also thank photographer Maurice Bruneau, Stacey Thidrickson (Associate Editor, Operations and Engagement, *Winnipeg Free Press*), Aimee Fortier (Manitoba Courts), and Andrea Gordon (Canadian Press) for their help with images.

We would also like to thank Brian Sinclair's family for their support of this project. They did not ask to have their brother and cousin die in the way that he did, and history has asked more of them than it ought to have. The Sinclair family's lawyer, Vilko Zbogar, was a critical resource, and we are grateful for his help. We thanks repositories for permission to reproduce photographs, and especially appreciate Maurice Bruneau and Karl Gomph for graciously providing images.

Much of this book was conceived over hip and delicious breakfasts at the Village Diner, located not far from where Brian Sinclair lived and ultimately died. On the walls of the café hung photographs of downtown Winnipeg taken in the 1960s and '70s, documenting a small slice of an ordinary Indigenous city. We hope that this book does justice to the rich and complex possibilities of Winnipeg, as well as to the structures of indifference that continue to cost us all so much, and some of us so much more than others.

NOTES

INTRODUCTION: THIRTY-FOUR HOURS

1   This group variously included other members involved at
    different junctures, including Janice Linton, Brenda Gunn,
    Leslie Spillett, Linda Diffey, and Christa Big Canoe. The
    BSWG is a group of Indigenous and non-Indigenous leaders,
    health advocates, physicians, nurses, legal experts, academics,
    and health researchers. The group formed to examine the role of
    racism in the death of Brian Sinclair and in the inquest that
    followed in order to highlight ongoing structural and systemic
    anti-Indigenous racism in our contemporary health and legal
    systems. So far, the activities of the BSWG have included
    establishing a cross-discipline collaborative discussion of
    systemic discrimination in the health care system. The BSWG
    wrote an op-ed for the *Winnipeg Free Press* (7 January 2014) to
    describe the problems its work is addressing. In April 2014, the
    BSWG held a public forum in Winnipeg that discussed the
    effects of discriminatory assumptions on a range of decisions
    made in health care, including diagnostic and treatment
    decisions. In September 2017 the BSWG organized an event
    with a presentation by Dr. Sherene Razack on how Brian
    Sinclair's death and inquest reflect common themes of
    indifference towards the unnatural deaths of Indigenous people
    in Canada. At this event, the BSWG released its interim report;
    a final report is anticipated.

2   Much of this work is discussed in Niigaan Sinclair, "Reconcilia-
    tion Lives Here: State of the Inner City Report 2016,"
    Canadian Centre for Policy Alternatives, available at https://

www.policyalternatives.ca/sites/default/files/uploads/
publications/Manitoba%20Office/2016/12/State_of_Inner_
City_Report_2016.pdf, accessed 12 June 2018.

3   "Brian Sinclair: Killed by Racism," available online at
    ignoredtodeathmanitoba.ca, accessed 8 May 2018.

4   This University of Manitoba Libraries LibGuide, "For Brian
    Sinclair," can be found at https://libguides.lib.umanitoba.ca/
    indigenoushealth/ForBrian, accessed 8 May 2018.

5   See Brian Sinclair Working Group, *Out of Sight: A Summary of
    Events Leading Up to Brian Sinclair's Death and the Inquest That
    Examined It and the Interim Recommendations of the Brian
    Sinclair Working Group* (Winnipeg 2017), available online at
    http://ignoredtodeathmanitoba.ca/index.php/2017/09/15/
    out-of-sight-interim-report-of-the-sinclair-working-group/, 4–8,
    accessed 4 January 2018.

6   See Provincial Court of Manitoba, "The Fatality Inquiries Act,
    in the Matter of Brian Lloyd Sinclair," 12 December 2014,
    http://www.manitobacourts.mb.ca/site/assets/files/1051/
    brian_sinclair_inquest_-_dec_14.pdf, accessed 4 January 2018
    (hereafter referred to as Final Report).

7   *Out of Sight*, 5–6.

8   Ann Laura Stoler, "Colonial Archives and the Arts of
    Governance," *Archival Science* 2 (2002): 87. Also see Ann Laura
    Stoler, *Along the Archival Grain: Epistemic Anxieties and
    Colonial Common Sense* (Princeton, NJ: Princeton University
    Press, 2010).

9   Audra Simpson, "Whither Settler Colonialism?" *Settler
    Colonial Studies* 6:4 (2016): 440.

10 Mary Jane Logan McCallum, "Condemned to Repeat? Settler
    Colonialism, Racism, and Canadian History Textbooks," in
    "Too Asian?" Racism, Privilege, and Post-Secondary Education, ed.
    Jeet Heer et al. (Toronto: Between the Lines, 2012), 67–79.

11 Sherene Razack, *Dying from Improvement: Inquests and
    Inquiries into Indigenous Deaths in Custody* (Toronto:
    University of Toronto Press, 2015), 194.

12   Patrick Wolfe, *Settler Colonialism and the Transformation of Anthropology: The Politics and Poetics of an Ethnographic Event* (London: Cassell, 1996), esp. Chapter 2.

13   Dina Gilio-Whitaker, "Settler Colonialism 101," on Thought-Co.com: https://www.thoughtco.com/american-settler-colonialism-4082454, accessed 12 June 2018.

14   Sherene H. Razack, "When Place Becomes Race," in *Race, Space, and the Law: Unmapping a White Settler Society*, ed. Sherene H. Razack (Toronto: Between the Lines," 2002), 3.

15   J. Kehaulani Kauanui, "A Structure, Not an Event": Settler Colonialism and Enduring Indigeneity," *Lateral: Journal of the Cultural Studies Association* 5:1 (Spring 2016).

16   http://www.statcan.gc.ca/daily-quotidien/171025/dq171025a-eng.pdf, accessed 26 January 2018.

17   Jean M. O'Brien, *Firsting and Lasting: Writing Indians Out of Existence in New England* (Minneapolis: University of Minnesota Press, 2010); Philip J. Deloria, *Indians in Unexpected Places* (Lawrence: University Press of Kansas, 2006); Susan Sleeper-Smith, Juliana Barr, Jean M. O'Brien, Nancy Shoemaker, and Scott Manning Stevens, eds., *Why You Can't Teach United States History without American Indians* (Chapel Hill: University of North Carolina Press, 2015); and Chris Andersen and Jean M. O'Brien, eds., *Sources and Methods in Indigenous Studies* (London: Routledge, 2016).

18   There is, at present, no formal mechanism to track Indigenous patients at the HSC; however, Dr. Marcia Anderson, Cree-Saulteaux physician, Medical Officer of Health with the Winnipeg Regional Health Authority, and assistant professor at the University of Manitoba, states that from her own perception, at any given time between 40 and 60 percent of the people using health care services provided by Winnipeg Regional Health Authority are Indigenous. Anderson, personal communication with McCallum, 30 March 2018. See also Susie Strachan, "Evolution of the Aboriginal Health Programs," which suggests that "up to 40 percent of urban hospital patients may be Indigenous" in Manitoba, at the Winnipeg Regional Health Authority website: http://www.wrha.mb.ca/healthinfo/

news/2016/160930-evolution-aboriginal-health-programs.php, accessed 5 April 2018.

19   Kimberlé Crenshaw, "Mapping the Margins: Intersectionality, Identity Politics, and Violence against Women of Color," *Stanford Law Review* 43:6 (July 1991): 1241–99.

20   "What Does Being Indigenous Mean?" http://www.cbc.ca/ news/canada/what-does-being-indigenous-mean-1.4172337, accessed 21 June 2017.

21   B. Allan and J. Smylie, *First Peoples, Second Class Treatment: The Role of Racism in the Health and Well-Being of Indigenous Peoples in Canada* (Toronto: Wellesley Institute, 2015); Samantha Loppie, Charlotte Reading, and Sarah de Leeuw, "Aboriginal Experiences with Racism and Its Impacts," Report for the National Collaborating Centre for Aboriginal Health, 2014, at: www.nccah-ccnsa.ca/ Publications/Lists/Publica- tions/Attachments/131/2014_07_09_FS_2426_RacismPart2_ ExperiencesImpacts_EN_Web.pdf, accessed 12 June 2018; Margo Greenwood, Sarah de Leeuw, and Nichole Marie Lindsay, eds., *Determinants of Indigenous People's Health: Beyond the Social*, 2nd edition (Toronto: Canadian Scholars Press, 2018); Charlotte Loppie Reading and Fred Wien, "Health Inequalities and Social Determinants of Aboriginal Peoples' Health," Report for the National Collaborating Centre for Aboriginal Health, 2009, at: https://www.ccnsa-nccah.ca/docs/determi- nants/RPT-HealthInequalities-Reading-Wien-EN.pdf, accessed 12 June 2018; Annette J. Browne, et al., "Enhancing Health Care Equity with Indigenous Populations: Evi- dence-based Strategies from an Ethnographic Study," *BMC Health Services Research* 16:544 (4 October 2016); and Yvonne Boyer, *Moving Aboriginal Health Forward: Discarding Canada's Legal Barriers* (Saskatoon: Purich Publishing Limited, 2015).

22   Mary Jane McCallum, "Rethinking History in Indigenous Health Research in Manitoba," unpublished paper delivered at the Critical Perspectives on Indigenous Histories and Health panel at the Native American and Indigenous Studies Association conference, Honolulu, Hawaii, May 2016; the San'yas Indigenous Cultural Safety Training program delivered by the Provincial Health Services Authority of British Columbia; the Manitoba Indigenous Cultural Safety Training

2011): 39–44; Fred. J. Shore, "The Emergence of the Metis Nation in Manitoba," in *Metis Legacy: A Metis Historiography and Annotated Bibliography*, ed. Lawrence J. Barkwell, Leah Dorion, and Darren R. Prefontaine (Winnipeg: Pemmican Publications, 2001), 75; "Memorable Manitobans: Curtis James Bird (1838–1876)" (Winnipeg: Manitoba Historical Society, updated October 2017), http://www.mhs.mb.ca/docs/people/bird_cj.shtml, accessed 12 June 2018.

19 See Shore, "The Emergence of the Metis," esp. 74–6.

20 Brad Milne, "The Historiography of Metis Land Dispersal, 1870–1890," *Manitoba History* 30 (Autumn 1995): 30–41.

21 See Adam Gaudry, "Metis," *Canadian Encyclopedia* (January 2009), https://www.thecanadianencyclopedia.ca/en/article/metis/, accessed 3 February 2018.

22 "Lord Selkirk's Treaty with the Indians, July 18, 1817," *Manitoba Pageant* 21:2 (Winter 1976), available at http://www.mhs.mb.ca/docs/pageant/21/lordselkirktreaty.shtml, accessed 16 February 2017.

23 See W.J. Healey, *Women of Red River: Being a Book Written from the Recollections of Women Surviving from the Red River Era* (Winnipeg: Women's Canadian Club, 1923), 19.

24 Heather Devine, *The People Who Own Themselves: Aboriginal Ethnogenesis in a Canadian Family, 1660–1900* (Calgary: University of Calgary Press, 2005); Robert Innes, "Elder Brother, the Law of the People, and Contemporary Kinship Practices of Cowessess First Nation Members: Conceptualizing Kinship in American Indian Studies Research," *American Indian Culture and Research Journal* 34:2 (2010): 27–46.

25 Aimée Craft, "Living Treaties, Breathing Research," *Canadian Journal of Women and the Law* 26:1 (2014), 3.

26 Ryan Eyford, *White Settler Reserve: New Iceland and the Colonization of the Canadian West* (Vancouver: UBC Press, 2016). Also see Sarah Carter, *Imperial Plots: Women, Land, and the Spadework of British Colonialism in the Canadian Prairies* (Winnipeg: University of Manitoba Press, 2016).

Program; and the Ontario Indigenous Cultural Safety Training Program. See also: Katerina Bezrukova et al., "A Meta-analytical Integration of Over 40 Years of Research on Diversity Training Evaluation," 2016, accessed 12 June 2018 from Cornell University, SHA School site: http://scholarship.sha.cornell.edu/articles/974; and M.M. Duguid and M.C. Thomas-Hunt, "Condoning Stereotyping? How Awareness of Stereotyping Prevalence Impacts Expression of Stereotypes," *Journal of Applied Psychology* 100:2 (March 2015): 343–59.

23 See the critique of this kind of analysis in Victor Ray, "*National Geographic* Acknowledges Its Racist Past, Then Steps on Its Message with a Cover Photo," *Washington Post*, 16 March 2018.

24 Greenwood, de Leeuw, Lindsay, and Reading, eds., *Determinants of Indigenous Peoples' Health: Beyond the Social*.

25 Mary Jane McCallum, "This Last Frontier: 'Isolation' and Aboriginal Health," *Canadian Bulletin of Medical History* 22:1 (2005): 103–120.

26 Jesse Thistle, "Vicarious Trauma: Collecting the Herd," *Active History* (3 November 2015), http://activehistory.ca/2015/11/vicarious-trauma-collecting-the-herd/, accessed 5 January 2018.

27 Zoe Todd, Twitter essay, 16 December 2017, https://twitter.com/ZoeSTodd/status/942059346736885761, accessed 4 April 2018.

28 See http://www.kanikanichihk.ca/, accessed 4 April 2018.

29 Mary Jane Logan McCallum, *Indigenous Women, Work, and History, 1940–1980* (Winnipeg: University of Manitoba Press, 2014), especially Introduction and Conclusion.

30 The timeline is based on the chronology outlined in *Out of Sight*, 12.

31 Final Report, 56.

32 Final Report, 53.

33 Final Report, 75.

34 Final Report, 21.

35 The family of Brian Sinclair maintained a website that kept the public updated on the legal proceedings surrounding the case,

including the inquest. It was called "ignoredtodeath.ca." While the original website is no longer maintained, there has been a concerted effort to, as much as possible, preserve significant, relevant documents at a new website: ignoredtodeathmanitoba.ca. The phrase "ignored to death" has been commonly used in media reporting on the issue.

CHAPTER ONE: THE CITY

1   Some of the archaeological work is summarized at https://humanrights.ca/about-museum/news/cmhr-releases-important-archaeology-findings-new-light-cast-historic-role-forks, accessed 2 February 2018.

2   See Catherine Flynn and E. Leigh Syms, "Manitoba's First Farmers," *Manitoba History* 31 (Spring 1996): 4–11.

3   Laura Peers, "The Ojibway, Red River, and the Forks, 1770–1870," in *The Forks and the Battle of Seven Oaks in Manitoba History*, ed. Robert Coutts and Richard Stuart (Winnipeg: Manitoba Historical Society, 1994).

4   Michael J. Witgen, *An Infinity of Nations: How the Native New World Shaped Early North America* (Philadelphia: University of Pennsylvania Press, 2012), 73.

5   See Adam Gaudry, "Metis Are a People, Not a Historical Process," *Canadian Encyclopedia,* http://www.thecanadianencyclopedia.ca/en/article/metis-are-a-people-not-a-historical-process/, accessed 8 May 2018.

6   Norma Hall, "Basic Stats for Red River, 1869–1870," in http://www.legislativeassemblyofassiniboia.ca/en/page/85/basic-stats-red-river-1869-1870, accessed 26 January 2018. Also see Gerhard Ens, *From Homeland to Hinterland: The Changing Worlds of the Red River Metis in the Nineteenth Century* (Toronto: University of Toronto Press, 1996).

7   Damon Ieremia Salesa, *Racial Crossings: Race, Intermarriage, and the Victorian British Empire* (Oxford: Oxford University Press, 2011).

8   See Denise Fuchs, "Embattled Notions: Constructions of Rupert's Land's Native Sons, 1760 to 1860," *Manitoba History* 44 (Autumn/Winter 2002–3): 10–17.

9   See Jennifer S.H. Brown, *Strangers in Blood: Fur Trade Company Families in Indian Country* (Vancouver: UBC Press, 1980), Chapter 8.

10 A.K. Isbister, "Suggestions for the Future Government of the Red River Territory, BNA," Appendix 2 in Barry Cooper, *Alexander Kennedy Isbister: A Respectable Critic of the Honourable Company* (Ottawa: Carleton University Press, 1988), 296, 300.

11 Adam Gaudry, "Fantasies of Sovereignty: Deconstructing British and Canadian Claims to Ownership of the Historic North-West," *NAIS* 3:1 (2016): 63.

12 See Norma Hall and Gerald Friesen, "Upper Fort Garry, 1869–70," 1, and notes 16 and 17, http://www.upperfortgarry.com/wp-content/uploads/2015/08/upper-fort-garry-1879-70.pdf, accessed 12 June 2018.

13 T.A. Heathcote, *British Field Marshals, 1736–1997: A Biographical Dictionary* (Barnsley, UK: Pen and Sword Books, 2012 [1999]).

14 From the Preface to the first edition, 1869. We thank Jill McConkey for this connection.

15 Louis Riel and A.D. Lepine to Lieutenant-Governor Morris, quoted in *Report of the Select Committee on the Causes of the Difficulties in the North-West Territory, 1869–70* (Ottawa: I.B. Taylor, 1874), 204.

16 See Allen Ronaghan, "James Farquharson—Agent and Agitator," *Manitoba History* 17 (Spring 1989).

17 Norma Hall, with Clifford P. Hall and Erin Verrier, *A History of the Legislative Assembly of Assiniboia/Le Conseil du Gouvernement Provisoire* (Winnipeg: Department of Aboriginal and Northern Affairs, 2010), 23.

18 See Gerald Friesen, *The Canadian Prairies: A History* (Toronto: University of Toronto Press, 1987), 195–6; Jérôme Marchildon, "The Story of Elzéar Goulet," *Manitoba History* 65 (Winter

27   George B. Elliot, *Winnipeg as It Is in 1874; And as It Was in 1860* (Winnipeg: Daily Free Press, n.d. [1874]): 22.

28   Nellie McClung, *Nellie McClung: The Complete Autobiography: Clearing in the West and the Stream Runs Fast*, ed. Veronica Strong-Boag and Michelle Lynn Rosa (Peterborough, ON: Broadview, 2003), 59.

29   Alan Artibise, *Winnipeg: A Social History of Urban Growth, 1874–1914* (Montreal: McGill-Queen's University Press, 1975), 130–1, Table 6.

30   Kurt Korneski, *Race, Nation, and Reform Ideology in Winnipeg, 1880s–1920s* (Madison, NJ: Fairleigh Dickinson University Press, 2015): 15.

31   E.J. Peters, "'Our City Indians': Negotiating the Meaning of First Nations Urbanization in Canada, 1945–1975," *Historical Geography* 30 (2002): 75.

32   Sarah Carter, *Aboriginal People and Colonizers of Western Canada to 1900* (Toronto: University of Toronto Press, 1999), 173.

33   Artibise, *Winnipeg*, 142, Table 12.

34   See David Burley, "Rooster Town: Winnipeg's Lost Metis Suburb, 1900–1960," *Urban History Review* 17:1 (Fall 2013): 3–25.

35   Megan Kozminski, "Empty-handed Constables and Notorious Offenders: Policing an Early Prairie City 'According to Order,'" in *Prairie Metropolis: New Essays on Winnipeg's Social History*, ed. Esyllt W. Jones and Gerald Friesen (Winnipeg: University of Manitoba Press, 2009), 56.

36   Jean H. Lagassé, *A Study of the Population of Indian Ancestry in Manitoba Undertaken by the Social and Economic Research Office: Main Report* (Winnipeg: Department of Agriculture and Immigration, 1959), 28.

37   Peters, "Our City Indians," 59.

38   Owen Toews, *Stolen City: Racial Capitalism and the Making of Winnipeg* (Winnipeg: ARP Books, forthcoming 2018), Chapter 2.

39   "Growth of Numbers Forcing Indians into Towns, Cities," *Winnipeg Free Press,* 24 January 1958.

40   See Peters, "Our City Indians," 78, Table 3.

41   Lagasse, *A Study*, 59, Table 2.

42   Mary Jane Norris and Stewart Clatworthy, "Aboriginal Mobility and Migration within Urban Canada: Outcomes, Factors, and Implications," in *Not Strangers in These Parts: Urban Aboriginal Peoples*, ed. David Newhouse and Evelyn Peters (Ottawa: Policy Research Initiative, 2003), 33, 37, 43.

43   Norris and Clatworthy, "Aboriginal Mobility and Migration," 50, 57, 61, 62.

44   Leslie Hall, "The Early History of the Winnipeg Indian and Metis Friendship Centre, 1951–1968," in Jones and Friesen, *Prairie Metropolis,* 223–41.

45   Jean H. Lagassé, "Community Development in Manitoba," *Human Organization* 20:4 (Winter 1961): 233.

46   Don N. McCaskill, "Migration, Adjustment, and Integration of the Indian into the Urban Environment" (PhD dissertation, Carleton University, 1970), 181.

47   Jim Silver, "Building a Path to a Better Future: Urban Aboriginal People," in *In Their Own Voices: Building Urban Aboriginal Communities*, ed. Jim Silver et al. (Halifax: Fernwood, 2006), 16.

48   Lagassé, *A Study*, 168.

49   McCaskill, "Migration, Adjustment, and Integration," 138.

50   Geoffrey Bernard Toews, "The Boons and Banes of Booze: The Liquor Trade in Rural Manitoba, 1929–1939," *Manitoba History* 50 (October 2005); see also Bartley Kives, "Alcohol: Lowering the Bar," *Winnipeg Free Press*, 19 January 2013.

51   Dale Barbour, "Drinking Together: The Role of Gender in Changing Manitoba's Liquor Laws in the 1950s," in Jones and Friesen, *Prairie Metropolis,* 181–2.

52   Warner Troyer, "Youth in Trouble: Crime Stems from Apathy," *Winnipeg Free Press,* 19 June 1962.

53 "Segregation in the Schools," *Winnipeg Free Press,* 13 December 1987.

54 Hall, "Winnipeg Indian and Metis Friendship Centre," 225.

55 Scott Rutherford, "Canada's Other Red Scare: Anicinabe Park Occupation and Indigenous Decolonization," in *The Hidden 1970s: Histories of Radicalism*, ed. Dan Berger (Rutgers, NJ: Rutgers University Press, 2010), 77–94.

56 Mary Jane Logan McCallum, "Winnipeg's History of Confronting Racism," *Winnipeg Free Press*, 2 April 2017.

57 See "Neeginan—A Future Native," in *History of the Winnipeg Indian and Metis Friendship Centre, 1958–1983* (Winnipeg: Indian and Metis Friendship Centre, 1983), 30, http://imfcentre.net/static/documents/25-year-history.pdf, 20 February 2017.

58 See Darrell Chippeway and Darryl Nepinak, "Preserving Aboriginal Institutional History in Winnipeg," 2013 video, https://www.policyalternatives.ca/multimedia/preserving-ab-original-institutional-history-winnipeg. See also John Loxley and Evelyn Peters, "Preserving the History of Aboriginal Institutional Development in Winnipeg: Research Driven by the Community," in *Community Based Participatory Research Methods: Practice and Transformative Change*, ed. Shauna McKinnon (Vancouver: UBC Press, forthcoming 2018). Sarah Story, "Offering our Gifts, Partnering for Change: Decoloniz-ing Experimentation in Winnipeg-based Settler Archives," MA thesis, University of Manitoba, 2017.

59 See John Einarson, "Rock and Racism," *Winnipeg Free Press*, 15 March 2015; Jesse Green and Vanda Fleury-Green, "Brown Town, Muddy Water" (Winnipeg: StrongFront TV, 2015).

60 Bonnie Devine, "Professional Native Indian Artists Inc., or the 'Indian Group of Seven,'" *Canadian Encyclopedia* (2015), http://www.thecanadianencyclopedia.ca/en/article/professional-na-tive-indian-artists-inc/, accessed 20 February 2018.

61 See Warren Cariou and Niigaanwewidam James Sinclair, eds., *Manitowapow: Aboriginal Writings from the Land of Water* (Winnipeg: Portage and Main Press, 2011).

62   For a summary, see http://www.cbc.ca/news/canada/manitoba/
      aboriginal-population-statistics-canada-1.4371222, accessed 21
      February 2018.

63   On Bowman's Metis identity, see Mary Agnes Welch, "The
      Metis Question: Defining the Uniquely Canadian People Who
      Founded Manitoba No Easy Task," *Winnipeg Free Press*, 14
      February 2015.

64   Kiera L. Ladner, "Do Star Indigenous Candidates and Party
      Platforms Translate into Votes?" in *Understanding the
      Manitoba Election: Campaigns, Participation, Issues, Place*, ed.
      Karine Levasseur, Andrea Rounce, Barry Ferguson, and Royce
      Koop (Winnipeg: University of Manitoba Press, 2016), 27–8.

65   Tom Carter, Chesya Polevychok, and Kurt Sargent, "Is
      Winnipeg's Aboriginal Population Ghettoized?" Research
      Highlight No. 2 (Winnipeg: Institute of Urban Studies,
      University of Winnipeg, December 2003).

66   Bartley Kives, "The 'Great Indigenous Divide': Winnipeg Stares
      into an Ethnic Chasm," *Guardian*, 21 October 2014; Nancy
      Macdonald, "Welcome to Winnipeg: Where Canada's Racism
      Problem Is at Its Worst," *Maclean's*, 22 January 2015.

67   Amnesty International, "Violence against Indigenous Women
      and Girls in Canada: A Summary of Amnesty International's
      Concerns and Call to Action," AmnestyInternational.ca, Febru-
      ary 2014, https://www.amnesty.ca/sites/amnesty/files/iwfa_
      submission_amnesty_international_february_2014_-_final.
      pdf, 2, accessed 12 June 2018.

68   Pamela Palmater, "Shining Light on the Dark Places:
      Addressing Police Racism and Sexualized Violence against
      Indigenous Women and Girls in the National Inquiry,"
      Canadian Journal of Women and the Law 23:2 (2016): 261.

69   Jaskiran Dhillon, *Prairie Rising: Indigenous Youth, Decoloniza-
      tion, and the Politics of Intervention* (Toronto: University of
      Toronto Press, 2017), 20.

CHAPTER TWO: THE HOSPITAL

1   See *Final Report of the Truth and Reconciliation Commission of Canada* (2015), available at http://www.trc.ca/websites/ trcinstitution/index.php?p=890, accessed 18 January 2018. See also *A Knock on the Door: The Essential History of Residential Schools from the Truth and Reconciliation Commission of Canada* (Winnipeg: University of Manitoba Press, 2015).

2   Jane Philpott, quoted in Jorge Barrera, "Indigenous Child Welfare Rates Creating 'Humanitarian Crisis' in Canada, says Federal Minister," http://www.cbc.ca/news/indigenous/ crisis-philpott-child-welfare-1.4385136, accessed 18 January 2018.

3   Peter Chura, "Report Flags Severe Overrepresentation of Aboriginals in Manitoba Jails," *Global News*, 16 October 2014, https://globalnews.ca/news/1618120/report-flags-se- vere-over-representation-of-aboriginals-in-manitoba-jails/, accessed 4 April 2018. The AJI also found that overrepresenta- tion in prisons was connected to a number of other inequities in the justice system; Indigenous people spend more time in pretrial detention, are more likely to be denied bail, and are more likely to be charged with multiple offences than non-Indigenous people who are accused. At the same time, the AJI also found that lawyers spend less time with Indigenous clients than they do with non-Indigenous clients. *Report of the Aboriginal Justice Inquiry of Manitoba* (Winnipeg: Aboriginal Justice Implementation Commission, November 1999), especially Volume 1, Chapter 4, http://www.ajic.mb.ca/ volume1/chapter4.html, accessed 12 June 2018.

4   In the last decade, while the population of white adults in Canadian prisons has declined, Indigenous incarceration rates have surged: for women, the rate rose 112 percent. Thirty-six percent of women and 25 percent of men sentenced to provincial and territorial custody are Indigenous. In 2016, *Maclean's* reported that "in some Prairie courtrooms, Indige- nous defendants now make up 85 percent of criminal caseloads." Nancy Macdonald, "Canada's Prisons Are the 'New Residential Schools," *Maclean's*, 18 February 2016, http://www.macleans.

ca/news/canada/canadas-prisons-are-the-new-residen-
tial-schools, accessed 12 June 2018.

5   In 1972, the Winnipeg General Hospital amalgamated with the
    Winnipeg Children's Hospital and the Winnipeg Rehabilita-
    tion Hospital to become the Health Sciences Centre.

6   "Hospital's New Critical Care Building Open to Public," *CBC
    News*, 11 January 2007, http://www.cbc.ca/news/canada/
    manitoba/hospital-s-new-critical-care-building-open-to-pub-
    lic-1.653658, accessed June 12 2018.

7   *Ann Thomas Callahan, Wapiskisiw Piyésís Iskwéw (White
    Birdwoman)* (Winnipeg: Health Sciences Centre), http://www.
    wrha.mb.ca/healthinfo/news/files/AnnThomasBio_Jan07.pdf.
    See also McCallum, *Indigenous Women, Work, and History*;
    Mary Jane Logan McCallum, *Twice As Good: A History of
    Aboriginal Nurses* (Ottawa: Aboriginal Nurses Association of
    Canada, 2007); and Leonard Monkman, "From Residential
    School to One of Manitoba's 1st Indigenous Nurses," *CBC
    News* (website), 18 March 2018, http://www.cbc.ca/news/
    indigenous/ann-thomas-callahan-indigenous-nurse-manito-
    ba-1.4577447, accessed 12 June 2018.

8   City of Winnipeg Historical Buildings Committee, "230
    Princess Street, Frost and Wood Warehouse," May 2002, http://
    www.winnipeg.ca/PPD/Documents/Heritage/ListHistorical-
    Resources/Princess-230-long.pdf, accessed 12 June 2018

9   Susan Jane Fisher, "Seeds from the Steppe: Mennonites,
    Horticulture, and the Construction of Landscapes on
    Manitoba's West Reserve, 1870–1950" (PhD thesis, University
    of Manitoba, 2017). See also Pamela Klassen and Joseph Wiebe,
    "'Reconciliation' with Indigenous People Is Comforting for
    Many Canadians, but Is a Christian Concept up to the Task?"
    Religion Dispatches, 19 March 2018, http://religiondispatches.
    org/reconciliation-with-indigenous-people-is-comfort-
    ing-for-many-canadians-but-is-a-christian-concept-up-to-the-
    task/, accessed 12 June 2018.

10 Tecumseh is the exception to the HBC's practice of naming
    streets around the hospital. Named before 1908 (previously it
    had been Silvia Street and Monkman Street; it later became
    Arlington), Tecumseh Street was next to Brant Street, both

likely named as a kind of flag of loyalty to Britain and commemoration of the War of 1812.

11 Harry Shave, "Little Street Honors Great Indian: The Origin of Tecumseh Street," *Winnipeg Free Press*, 3 August 1963, 18.

12 Robin Jarvis Brownlie, "The Co-optation of Tecumseh: The War of 1812 and Racial Discourse in Upper Canada," *Journal of the CHA,* 2012, New Series 23(1): 39–63; and Sean Carleton, "Rebranding Canada with Comics: Canada 1812: Forged in First and the Continuing Co-optation of Tecumseh," *ActiveHistory. ca*, 9 April 2014, http://activehistory.ca/papers/history-papers-15/, accessed 12 June 2018.

13 Harry Shave, "Streets Named before 1908," from the Manitoba Historical Society website, http://www.mhs.mb.ca/docs/ winnipegstreets/#p, accessed 12 June 2018.

14 For example, Sherbrook Street was originally named Mulligan after James Mulligan, who operated a ferry across the Assiniboine River near Misericordia Hospital. It was renamed Sherbrook in 1897. Mulligan came to Red River in 1848 with a contingent of British troops who were promised land in the colony after military service. His plot of land ran from the river to Portage, Furby to Maryland. Mulligan served as a police officer and was imprisoned by Louis Riel in 1869. Notre Dame was named in 1891 for a Catholic girls' school on the street, which later moved to Academy Road. William Street was named in 1893 for William Ross, son of Alexander Ross. William was born in the Columbia River area in 1825 and moved with his family when Alexander decided to retire to Red River. William was appointed Sheriff of Assiniboia in 1851 and in 1855 became the first postmaster of the Red River settlement. He lived in Ross House for two years and died in May 1856. His mother was Sarah Ross (1798–1884), daughter of an Okanagan chief. She married Alexander according to the "custom of the country" in 1812 and in an Anglican church in 1828. She "seldom appeared in public," but was a well-known figure in the community, serving as "a link between Indian tribal life, the mixed-bloods, and the new white communities of traders." See Laurenda Daniells, "Sally (Sarah) Ross," *Dictionary of Canadian Biography XI (1881–1890)*, http://www.biographi.ca/ en/bio.php?BioId=39933, accessed 12 June 2018.

15   Sarah was an issuer of this grant (it predated the Dominion Lands Act).

16   Norma J. Hall, ed., "McNab," *Mothers of the Resistance 1869–1870: Red River Metis Genealogies*, https://resistance-mothers.wordpress.com/about/mcnab/, accessed 12 June 2018.

17   "The Bazaar," *Manitoban and Northwest Herald*, 9 August 1873, 3; "Card of Thanks," *Manitoba Free Press*, 16 August 1873, 5.

18   *Manitoba Free Press*, 25 July 1874, 5.

19   Todd Lamirande and the Louis Riel Institute, "Annie McDermot (Bannatyne)," *Sessional Papers* (Manitoba: Legislative Assembly, The Treasurer, In account with the Winnipeg General Hospital from 14 May 1875 to 31 December 1875), 5, http://www.metismuseum.ca/media/db/07426, accessed 12 June 2018.

20   See also Norma J. Hall, "Anne 'Annie' McDermont Bannatyne," https://hallnjean2.wordpress.com/the-red-river-resistence/women-and-the-resistance/annie-mcdermot-bannatyne/, accessed 8 May 2018.

21   "The Bazaar," *Manitoban and Northwest Herald*, 9 August 1873, 3.

22   Adele Perry, *Aqueduct: Colonialism, Resources, and the Histories We Remember* (Winnipeg: ARP Books, 2016).

23   Ian Carr and Robert E. Beamish, *Manitoba Medicine*: *A Brief History* (Winnipeg: University of Manitoba Press, 1999), 31.

24   Department of Indian Affairs Annual Reports show that First Nations people were permitted treatment at the Winnipeg General Hospital until at least the early 1920s; and at St. Boniface Hospital until the early 1930s.

25   They even made health care services available to settlers, especially prior to the establishment of the colonial medical institutions. Maureen Lux, *Medicine That Walks: Disease, Medicine, and the Canadian Plains Native People, 1880–1940* (Toronto: University of Toronto Press, 2001), 19; Kristin Burnett, *Taking Medicine: Women's Healing Work and Colonial Contact in Southern Alberta, 1880–1930* (Vancouver: UBC Press, 2010); Laurie Meijer Drees, *Healing Histories: Stories*

from Canada's Indian Hospitals (Edmonton: University of Alberta Press, 2013); and Mary-Ellen Kelm, *Colonizing Bodies: Aboriginal Health and Healing in British Columbia, 1900–1950* (Vancouver: UBC Press, 1999), 129.

26 Eyford, *White Settler Reserve*, Chapter 4.

27 David A. Stewart, "The Red Man and the White Plague," *Canadian Medical Association Journal* 35 (1936): 674.

28 Maureen K. Lux, *Separate Beds: A History of Indian Hospitals in Canada, 1920s–1980s* (Toronto: University of Toronto Press, 2016), 19.

29 P.H. Bryce, *Report on the Indian Schools of Manitoba and the North West Territories* (Ottawa: Government Printing Bureau), 28. Available at http://peel.library.ualberta.ca/bibliography/3024.html, accessed 5 June 2018.

30 Kelm, *Colonizing Bodies,* 113; and Department of Indian Affairs, Annual Report, 1927, 10.

31 Lux, *Separate Beds.* For more on racially segregated tuberculosis case findings, treatment, and rehabilitation programs in Manitoba, see McCallum's research website "Indigenous Histories of Tuberculosis in Manitoba, 1930–1970," https://indigenoustbhistories.wordpress.com, accessed 8 May 2018.

32 Lux, *Separate Beds,* 6; see also James Daschuk, *Clearing the Plains: Disease, Politics of Starvation, and the Loss of Aboriginal Life* (Regina: University of Regina Press, 2013), Robert Alexander Innes, "Historians and Indigenous Genocide in Saskatchewan," 21 June 2018, https://shekonneechie.ca/2018/06/21/historians-and-indigenous-genocide-in-saskatchewan.

33 Maureen Lux, "Indian Hospitals in Canada," *Canadian Encyclopedia,* http://www.thecanadianencyclopedia.ca/en/article/indian-hospitals-in-canada/, accessed 4 June 2018.

34 Paul Hackett, "'That Will Not Be Done Again': The Fort Alexander Preventorium and the Fight against Tuberculosis in Indian Residential Schools, 1937–1939," *Native Studies Review* 21:1 (2012): 1–41; "Pine Falls Hospital" and "Fort Alexander

Hospital," Library and Archives Canada, RG 29 Volume 2931 File 851-1-x200 pt. 4; Lux, *Separate Beds*, 15–17.

35   Lux, *Separate Beds*, 15.

36   "Pine Falls Hospital" and "Fort Alexander Hospital," Library and Archives Canada, RG 29 Volume 2931 File 851-1-x200 pt 4; Lux, *Separate Beds*, 15–17.

37   Personal communication with Bella Malo, 14 and 20 June 2018.

38   "Pine Falls Hospital," 3–4, n.d. (visited 25 February 1960), Library and Archives Canada, RG 29 Volume 2931 File 851-1-x200 pt 4.

39   "Fort Alexander Hospital," 2, n.d. (visited 25 February 1960), Library and Archives Canada, RG 29 Volume 2931 File 851-1-x200 pt 4..

40   Lux, *Separate Beds*, 131 and 154.

41   Heidi Bohaker and Franca Iacovetta, "Making Aboriginal People 'Immigrants Too': A Comparison of Citizenship Programs for Newcomers and Indigenous Peoples in Postwar Canada, 1940s–1960s," *Canadian Historical Review* 90:3 (September 2009): 461.

42   *Healing and Hope: A History of Health Sciences Centre Winnipeg* (Winnipeg: Health Sciences Centre Winnipeg, 2009), 148.

43   Nichole Margaret Marie Riese, "Perceptions of Care: Aboriginal Patients at the Winnipeg Health Sciences Centre" (MSc thesis, University of Manitoba 2001), 54; and "No Criminal Intent; Plenty of Shame," *Winnipeg Free Press*, 9 September 2017.

44   It was estimated that even ten years later, in 2001, Indigenous people still comprised less than 1 percent of the hospital's workforce. Riese, "Perceptions of Care," x.

45   McCallum, "This Last Frontier."

46   Jessica Kolopenuk, "Pathological Kinships: Blood, DNA, and Tuberculosis Research Among Indigenous Peoples in Canada," unpublished paper presented at the Manitoba-Ontario-Minnesota-Saskatchewan History of Medicine Conference, Winnipeg, September 2017; and "Scientific Fragility," unpublished paper

presented at the Native American and Indigenous Studies Association Conference, Los Angeles, 2018.

47 Linda Diffey and Barry Lavallee, "Is Cultural Safety Enough? Confronting Racism to Address Inequities in Indigenous Health," *OFED News* 2 (2016),, 2–3, accessed 6 June 2018 at: https://umanitoba.ca/faculties/health_sciences/medicine/education/ed_dev/media/June10-OEFD_Newsletter_2016_spring.pdf.

48 See "Information Sheet: Jordan's Principle: Summary of Orders from the Canadian Human Rights Tribunal," https://fncaringsociety.com/sites/default/files/Summary%20of%20Jordan%27s%20Principle%20Orders%20%282018%20update%29.pdf, accessed 8 May 2018.

49 See Dan Lett, "Jordan's Principle Remains in Limbo," *Canadian Medical Association Journal* 12 (2 December 2008), http://www.cmaj.ca/content/179/12/1256, accessed 12 June 2018.

CHAPTER THREE: BRIAN SINCLAIR

1 Dr. Janet Smylie identified individual acts of bias and stereotyping and has documented ongoing anti-Indigenous racism in the health care system. Dr. Catherine Cook pointed to the ways in which historical racism and exclusion continue to shape Indigenous people's access to health care.

2 For a summary, see Brian Sinclair Working Group, "Ignored to Death," and see http://ignoredtodeathmanitoba.ca/ for the transcripts and related documents.

3 Submission of counsel for the Sinclair family to the Honourable Timothy J. Preston, 18 February 2014, quoted in full at "Brian Sinclair's Family Loses Confidence, Pulls Out of Inquest," http://www.cbc.ca/news/canada/manitoba/brian-sinclair-s-family-loses-confidence-pulls-out-of-inquest-1.2541167, accessed 3 March 2018.

4 Testimony of Esther Joyce Grant, 6 August 2013, Consolidated Sinclair Inquest Transcripts (hereafter referred to as Consolidated Transcripts), found at https://www.dropbox.com/s/

e8mockdl1o5ywlz/Sinclair%20inquest%20transcripts%20
-%20consolidated.pdf?dl=0, accessed 12 June 2018: 40–42.

5   See, for instance, Bonita Lawrence, *"Real" Indians and Others:
    Mixed-Blood Urban Native Peoples and Indigenous Nationhood*
    (Vancouver: UBC Press, 2004); Martin J. Cannon, "First
    Nations Citizenship: An Act to Amend the Indian Act (1985)
    and the Accommodation of Sex Discrimination Policy,"
    Canadian Review of Social Policy 56 (2006): 40–71; Janet
    Silman, ed., *Enough Is Enough: Aboriginal Women Speak Out*
    (Toronto: Women's Press, 1987).

6   See Megan Furi and Jill Wherrett, "Indian Status and Band
    Membership Issues," 2003, https://lop.parl.ca/content/lop/
    researchpublications/bp410-e.htm#achangestx, accessed 11
    March 2018.

7   Consolidated Transcripts, 61–3.

8   Chelsea Vowel, *Indigenous Writes: A Guide to First Nations,
    Metis, and Inuit Issues in Canada* (Winnipeg: HighWater Press,
    2016), 121–34.

9   Testimony of Esther Joyce Grant, Consolidated Transcripts, 42.

10 See Peggy Martin-McGuire, "First Nations Land Surrenders on
    the Prairies, 1896–1911" (Ottawa: Indian Claims Commission,
    September 1998), xiii.

11 Sarah Carter, "They Would Not Give Up One Inch of It': The
    Rise and Demise of St Peter's Reserve, Manitoba," in Alan
    Lester and Zoe Laidlaw, eds., *Indigenous Communities and
    Settler Dispossession* (London: Palgrave, 2015), 173–93.

12 Historic Sites of Manitoba: Pine Falls Paper Mill (Power-
    view-Pine Falls) at the Manitoba Historical Society website:
    http://www.mhs.mb.ca/docs/sites/pinefallspapermill.shtml,
    accessed 8 March 2018.

13 See McCallum, *Indigenous Women, Work, and History*, Chapter
    1.

14 Raven Sinclair, "Identity Lost and Found: Lessons from the
    Sixties Scoop," *First Peoples Child and Family Review* 3:1
    (2007): 66.

15 Testimony of Esther Joyce Grant, Consolidated Transcripts, 64–7.

16 On the history of Indigenous children and foster care in these years, see Veronica Strong-Boag, *Fostering Nation? Canada Confronts Its History of Childhood Disadvantage* (Waterloo: Wilfrid Laurier University Press, 2011), 100–5.

17 Testimony of Esther Joyce Grant, Consolidated Transcripts, 50–2.

18 Consolidated Transcripts, 7. See also http://www.gov.mb.ca/publictrustee/, accessed 18 March 2018.

19 See http://www.questhealth.ca/Accommodations.html, accessed 19 March 2018.

20 See https://siloam.ca/, accessed 19 March 2018.

21 Testimony of Ken McGhie, 6 August 2013, Consolidated Transcripts, 70–1.

22 Testimony of Darwin Ironstand, Consolidated Transcripts, 42. See also the testimony of Clarissa Immaculata.

23 See, for instance, the testimony of D.G. Connolly, Consolidated Transcripts, 89.

24 Testimony of Ken McGhie, Consolidated Transcripts, 67.

25 Testimony of Diane Kubas, Consolidated Transcripts, 35.

26 Provincial Court of Manitoba, "The Fatality Inquiries Act in the Matter of Brian Lloyd Sinclair" (12 December 2014), 6.

27 Testimony of Laura Johnson, Consolidated Transcripts, 115.

28 Testimony of Howard Nepinak, Consolidated Transcripts, 69–99.

29 Testimony of Leslie Spillett, Consolidated Transcripts, 35.

30 Robert Alexander Innes and Kim Anderson, "Introduction: Who Is Walking with Our Brothers?" in *Indigenous Men and Masculinities: Legacies, Identities, Regeneration*, ed. Robert Alexander Innes and Kim Anderson (Winnipeg: University of Manitoba Press, 2015), 4.

31 See, for instance, Lindor Reynolds, "Patient's Demise Raises Troubling Questions," *Winnipeg Free Press*, 24 September 2008; "Brian Sinclair Dead for Hours in Hospital ER, Inquest Told," *CBC News*, 7 August 2013, http://www.cbc.ca/news/canada/manitoba/brian-sinclair-dead-for-hours-in-hospital-er-inquest-told-1.1359805, accessed 12 June 2018; and "'This Man's Problems Were Self-Inflicted': Doctor Says Man Who Died Waiting in Winnipeg ER for 34 Hours Partly Responsible," *National Post*, 8 August 2013.

32 For discussions of Indigenous people and homelessness in Canada and the settler colonial world, see Evelyn J. Peters and Julia Christensen, eds., *Indigenous Homelessness: Perspectives from Canada, Australia, and New Zealand* (Winnipeg: University of Manitoba Press, 2016).

33 Testimony of Diane Kubas, 22 August 2013, Consolidated Transcripts, 130.

34 Testimony of J.J. O'Donovan, 27 August 2013, Consolidated Transcripts, 489.

35 Testimony of K.L. Ranson, 13 August 2013, Consolidated Transcripts, 51.

36 Roxanne Dunbar-Ortiz and Dina Gilio-Whitaker, "What's Behind the Myth of Native American Alcoholism," *Pacific Standard*, 10 October 2016.

37 Vowel, *Indigenous Writes,* 151–6.

38 Also see Testimony of J.J. O'Donovan, 27 August 2013, Consolidated Transcripts, 56.

39 Testimony of J.J. O'Donovan, 26 August 2013, Consolidated Transcripts, 96–7.

40 Testimony of J.J. O'Donovan, 27 August 2013, Consolidated Transcripts, 53.

41 "This Man's Problems Were Self-Inflicted," *National Post*, 8 August 2013; "Doctor's Email about Brian Sinclair Sparks Criticism," *CBC News*, 9 August 2013, http://www.cbc.ca/news/canada/manitoba/doctor-s-email-about-brian-sinclair-sparks-criticism-1.1341549, accessed 23 March 2018.

42   Testimony of T. Balachandra, 6 August 2013, Consolidated Transcripts, 118, and 7 August 2013, Consolidated Transcripts, 8, 12, 36–7.

43   Final Report, 23.

44   Razack, *Improved to Death*, 139.

45   Mandi Gray, "Pathologizing Indigenous Suicide: Examining the Inquest into the Deaths of C.J. and C.B. at the Manitoba Youth Centre," *Studies in Social Justice* 10:1 (2016): 81.

46   Tanya Talaga, *Seven Fallen Feathers: Racism, Death, and Hard Truths in a Northern City* (Toronto: House of Anansi, 2017).

47   Razack, *Improved to Death,* 203.

CONCLUSION

1   Carmela Murdocca, "'A Matter of Time and a Matter of Place': Colonial Inquiries and the Politics of Testimony," *Law, Culture, and the Humanities* 13:1 (2017): 141.

2   Opening Remarks of William Olsen, 6 August 2013, Consolidated Transcripts, 16.

3   Final Report, 28 and 64.

4   Testimony of T. Balachandra, 7 August 2013, Consolidated Transcripts, 67.

5   Testimony of T. Balachandra, 7 August 2013, Consolidated Transcripts, 67.

6   Testimony of Wendy Krongold, 10 October 2013, Consolidated Transcripts, 97.

7   Kurtz et al., "Silence of Voice: An Act of Structural Violence: Urban Aboriginal Women Speak Out about Their Experiences with Health Care," *Journal of Aboriginal Health* 4:1 (2008): 53–63; S. Tang and A.J. Browne, "'Race Matters': Racialization and Egalitarian Discourses Involving Aboriginal People in the Canadian Health Care Context," *Ethnicity and Health* 13:2 (2008): 109–27; Browne et al., "Access to Primary Care from the Perspective of Aboriginal Patients at an Urban Emergency Department," *Qualitative Health Research* 21:3 (2011): 333–48;

B. Allan and J. Smylie, *First Peoples, Second Class Treatment: The Role of Racism in the Health and Well-Being of Indigenous Peoples in Canada* (Toronto: Wellesley Institute, 2015).

8   Janet Smylie, quoted in Emily Blake, "People 'dying unnecessarily' because of racial bias in Canada's health-care system, researcher says," *CBC News*, 3 July 2018, https://www.cbc.ca/news/canada/north/health-care-racial-bias-north-1.4731483, accessed 10 July 2019.

9   Truth and Reconciliation Commission of Canada, "Calls to Action," 2015, http://www.trc.ca/websites/trcinstitution/File/2015/Findings/Calls_to_Action_English2.pdf , accessed 10 July 2019, 2–3. We thank editor Jill McConkey for her framing of this point.

10 Tania Dick, "'It Has Eaten a Hole in My Heart': Indigenous Nurses Recall Systemic Racism with Life-or-Death Consequences," interview on *The Current (CBC News)*, 2 March 2018.

11 Lux, *Separate Beds*.

12 http://aptnnews.ca/2017/09/22/stolo-nation-woman-allegedly-told-to-leave-hospital-after-suffering-multiple-fractures/; http://www.cbc.ca/news/canada/montreal/muhc-indigenous-woman-kimberly-gloade-1.4221827; http://www.cbc.ca/news/canada/montreal/muhc-investigation-indigenous-women-1.4560383; all accessed 23 March 2018.

13 *Our Women and Girls Are Sacred: Interim Report of the National Inquiry into Missing and Murdered Indigenous Women and Girls* (Ottawa: Government of Canada, 2017), 8.

14 Cameron MacLean, "Senior Corrections Officer Made Call to Shackle Errol Greene during Seizures, Inquest Told," *CBC News*, 31 January 2018, http://www.cbc.ca/news/canada/manitoba/errol-greene-inquest-corrections-officer-1.4512850, accessed 25 March 2018.

15 Steve Lambert, "Winnipeg Man's Death in Remand Centre Should 'Expose the Truth' about Inmate Treatment, Widow Says," *Globe and Mail*, 28 January 2018, https://www.theglobeandmail.com/news/national/winnipeg-mans-death-in-remand-centre-should-expose-the-truth-about-inmate-treatment-widow-says/article37760315/, accessed 23 March 2018.

16 Gina Starblanket and Dallas Hunt, "How the Death of Colten Boushie Became Recast as the Story of a Knight Protecting His Castle," 13 February 2018, https://www.theglobeandmail.com/opinion/how-the-death-of-colten-boushie-became-recast-as-the-story-of-a-knight-protecting-his-castle/article37958746/, accessed 23 March 2018.

17 See Kathleen Harris, "Liberals Review Jury Selection Process after Boushie Case Uproar," *CBC News*, 12 February 2018, http://www.cbc.ca/news/politics/jury-selection-diversity-indigenous-1.4531792, accessed 25 March 2018; Ken Roach, "Ending Peremptory Challenges in Jury Selection Is a Good First Step," *Ottawa Citizen,* 2 April 2018, accessed at http://ottawacitizen.com/opinion/columnists/roach-ending-peremptory-challenges-in-jury-selection-is-a-good-first-step, 4 April 2018.

18 Robert Jago, "In the Trial of Gerald Stanley, an All-white Jury Runs from Justice," 10 February 2018, https://www.mediaindigena.com/in-the-trial-of-gerald-stanley-an-all-white-jury-ran-from-justice/, accessed 23 March 2018.

19 Robert Innes quoted in Jason Warick, "No Hate Speech Charges Laid in Colten Boushie Case," 18 February 2018, http://www.cbc.ca/news/canada/saskatoon/colten-boushie-hate-speech-charges-1.3989413, accessed 4 April 2018.

ILLUSTRATION CREDITS

---

1. Inquest Exhibit 63, courtesy Manitoba Courts.
2. Inquest Exhibit 15. With thanks to Vilko Zgobar. **3.** G. Kemp, Peter Winkworth Collection of Canadiana, Library and Archives Canada, acc. R9226-3441, item 3441, e000756700. **4.** William James Topley Studio, Library and Archives Canada, acc. 1936-270, item 1879, PA-009839. **5.** Wikimedia Commons, https://commons.wikimedia.org/w/index.php?title=File:Numbered-Treaties-Map.svg&oldid=292751115. **6.** Map by Eric Leinberger. Originally published in Ryan Eyford, *White Settler Reserve: New Iceland and the Colonization of the Canadian West* (Vancouver: UBC Press, 2016). Used with permission. **7.** Lyall Commercial Photo Co., Library and Archives Canada, acc. 1966-094 NPC, item 27637, PA-030060. **8.** "Growth of Numbers Forcing Indians into Towns, Cities," *Winnipeg Free Press*, 24 January 1958. **9.** University of Manitoba Archives and Special Collections, *Winnipeg Tribune* Photo Collection, PC 18/7150/18-6309-007.

10. Department of Indian Affairs and Northern Development, Library and Archives Canada, acc. 1976-281 NPC, item 3138, PA-202475. **11.** Winnipeg Regional Health Authority. **12.** C.C. Chataway's Map of Winnipeg (Western Map Company, 1919). North East Winnipeg Historical Society. **13.** *Manitoba Free Press*, Saturday, 28 May 1910, p. 24. **14.** Notman & Sandham Studio Collection, McCord Museum, no. 77678. **15.** Medical Campus Architecture Collection, University of Manitoba College of Medicine Archives, CA 046A. **16.** Photo courtesy of Bella Malo, née Guimond, from Shirley Lavallee's album. **17.** *Canada's Health and Welfare*, Indian and Northern Health Services Supplement No. 38 (February 1961). **18.** Photographer Unknown, Sam Waller Museum, PP2002.23.87. **19.** Rob Mathieson, Margaret Smith, Aboriginal Services/Native Services, University of Manitoba College of Medicine Archives. **20.** Jan McLaren, Quality Support, Aboriginal Services, University of Manitoba College of Medicine Archives. **21.** Department of Indian and Northern Affairs, Library and Archives Canada, acc. 1967-281, item 06-02-07-00, PA-185653. **22.** University of Manitoba Archives and Special Collections, *Winnipeg Tribune* Photo Collection, PC 18/4642/18-3834-012. **23.** Karl Gomph, with thanks to Vilko Zgobar. **24.** Map by Weldon Hiebert. Contains information licensed under the

Open Government Licence – Canada. **25.** Boris Minkevich, *Winnipeg Free Press*, 6 August 2013. **26.** University of Manitoba Archives and Special Collections, *Winnipeg Tribune* Photo Collection, PC 89-095-006. **27.** Courtesy of Maurice Bruneau.

INDEX